A Colour Atlas of
DIAGNOSIS AFTER RECENT INJURY

P.S. London
MBE, CStJ, FRCS, MFOM, FACEM (Hon)
Honorary Consulting Surgeon
The Birmingham Accident Hospital

Wolfe Medical Publications Ltd

Copyright © P.S. London, 1990
Published by Wolfe Medical Publications Ltd, 1990
Printed by W.S. Cowell Ltd, Ipswich, England
ISBN 0 7234 1520 X

A CIP catalogue record for this book is available from the British Library.

This book is one of the titles in the series of Wolfe Medical Atlases, a series that brings together the world's largest systematic published collection of diagnostic colour photographs.

For a full list of Wolfe Medical Atlases, plus forthcoming titles and details of our surgical, dental and veterinary Atlases, please write to Wolfe Publishing Ltd, 2-16 Torrington Place, London WC1E 7LT, England.

Contents

Acknowledgements

The illustrations in this volume have been collected over a period of nearly 30 years, and for this reason some of the equipment and methods of treatment shown may be out of date. However, the appearance of injuries and their effects have changed very little over a much longer period.

For collecting the illustrations I have depended heavily on the ever-willing collaboration of the photographers at the Birmingham Accident Hospital, particularly Mr N.R. Gill, Miss D. Moore (now Mrs Scott) and Mr A. Turner, who not only attended promptly and waited patiently on many occasions but even stayed on duty or came into the hospital outside working hours when cases of special interest were involved. This atlas can fairly be regarded as a testament to their loyalty and sense of service. I also thank Mr and Mrs Robert Hopwood for their assistance in the preparation of the slides used and Mr G.D. Wood, MDS, MSc, FDS, RCPSG (5) and Update-Siebert Publications Limited for granting permission to reproduce illustrations from their publications (**387, 388, 400, 410, 411**), Mr H. Proctor (**82**), Mr J.E.M. Smith (**91**), Mr T.R. Fisher (**136, 212**), Mr E.K. Alpar (**137**), Mr J.H. Hicks (**205**), Butterworths and Mr D.J.W. McMinn (**298**), Mr D. Jaffray (**338**).

I am also grateful to my surgical colleagues for permission to photograph their patients or for providing me with copies of their photographs. I can only hope that those that recognise illustrations but whose courtesy has not been formally acknowledged, will look indulgently on my oversight or poor memory—they deserve better.

Finally, I express my gratitude to Miss Amaryllis Bigley for her cheerful willingness and application in the conversion of my tortured draft into an immaculate typescript.

Foreword

The importance of the history in the process of diagnosis is well known. However, it is not always possible to obtain such history, with the result that a doctor's, nurse's or first aider's primary evidence that injury has occurred may be what is seen. Such evidence may be obvious but there are occasions when it is slight, vague or subtle with the result that it goes unrecognised for what it is, unless the observer knows how to interpret it.

This atlas could well have been titled 'Ho ho! Lesions explained': the term may seem flippant but it is striking and likely to be remembered as a warning that seeming trivia must on occasion arouse suspicion as to their cause, as in 'Ho ho! What have we here?'

The term 'emergency room' is of American origin and is synonymous with the British term 'Accident and Emergency Department'.

To those at the 'sharp end' of accident services

1 Introduction

The plan of this atlas is based on the method of examination of a severely injured and perhaps unconscious casualty in that it deals systematically with the injured person from head to foot and back and front.

Although the book is not concerned with treatment as such, there are occasions when the last step in diagnosis (exploration) is the first step in treatment and one aspect cannot be adequately considered without mentioning the other. There are also circumstances in which treatment will be defective unless the therapeutic implications of the injury to be treated are understood thoroughly. The outcome of treatment is given when it has a bearing on the process of diagnosis.

Each section deals first, in appropriate circumstances, with what is visible from the front, then what can be seen at the sides and on such upper and lower surfaces as exist, and then with the back. The illustrations have been presented as they would appear to an examiner standing beside a bed or couch, or having the patient standing up or sitting down.

The classification of the signs of injury into bruises and grazes, wounds, swelling, deformity and posture, and, in some cases, infection, is to some extent artificial in that they may occur separately or together. Furthermore, similar signs may have different causes and vice versa. The justification is that these signs provide evidence that should be noted and interpreted in the light of the circumstances of injury and such physical signs as may be detected.

Most victims of an accident have sustained only one injury and the injured person can give more or less a helpful summary of the circumstances and the resulting symptoms. Even so, the data provided may be, quite unintentionally, misleading and require an experienced observer to base diagnosis, or at least suspicion, on what he/she finds and then proceed to put the suspicion to the test by careful examination by clinical and other means.

This may be exemplified by the way in which a teacher on occasion takes one look at a patient and tells an astonished pupil (and patient) what happened and names the symptoms.

This atlas offers to students and practitioners of medicine, nursing, first aid at the more advanced levels of ambulance services, and to simulators of injury, the visible evidence that should at least arouse suspicion and, in some cases, may justify a confident diagnosis of the cause.

General examination of the seriously injured

Modern methods have brought to the care of the seriously injured a remarkable degree of accuracy in diagnosis and success in treatment. However, they are not universally available and, in some cases, when they are available, they are not practicable. Careful clinical examination is always possible; its value should not be underestimated even in the best-equipped hospitals.

The successful use of elaborate methods of investigation depends upon good team work. However, there is a danger that the individual members of the diagnostic and therapeutic team will concentrate upon individual tasks; as a result the patient will become subdivided into perhaps half-a-dozen fields of interest, while needles and tubes of various sorts are inserted and various samples are withdrawn, and dressings and splints are applied. Such concentration of effort may be essential to the survival of the injured person, but it can lead to a failure to consider the patient as a whole and piece together scattered signs into a usefully informative picture. Whenever possible, one member of the team should observe the proceedings closely and be prepared to point out noteworthy evidence, errors and omissions. This is best done by someone with wide experience but such a person may well not be available on the spot during the hectic few minutes after a seriously injured person is admitted to a reception and emergency room.

Responsibility for knowledgeable interpretation of noteworthy signs does not lie solely on the medical staff on duty. In the case of serious injuries, nurses undressing the casualty may be the first to observe signs that should be drawn to a doctor's attention. In the ordinary emergency room, an experienced nurse has much to offer a young doctor whose self-confidence may outweigh his/her knowledge or judgement, or who is in doubt about whether or not to disturb a senior's slumbers.

The increasingly ready availability of accurate diagnostic tools is too easily and too often thought by junior staff to have reduced the need for detailed clinical examination. This is an extremely dangerous assumption. Inadequate clinical examination followed by misinterpretation of radiological or other findings can have disastrous results. In other cases the need for prompt action to identify and to mitigate a threat to life has to be based on physical signs alone; an example is a rapidly expanding pneumothorax.

The best experience in handling and coping with injuries comes from having plenty of patients to study and ready access to an experienced teacher. This atlas is no substitute for either but it does offer an introduction to the important art of recognising what matters and knowing how to interpret it, and it may help to promote an understanding of anatomy that is sadly deficient among junior hospital staff. For this reason it can be helpful to be able to refer readily to textbooks or to models, and particularly to cross sections that may be available as diagrams or as computed tomograms.

2 The head and neck

Bruises and grazes

The alarming appearances of a patient on arrival at hospital can sometimes be attributed more to the amount of blood and dirt that is visible than to damaged tissues.

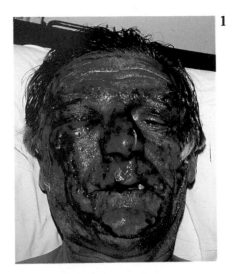

The results of cleansing

1 Appearance of a man on admission to hospital after being attacked in the street.

2 Appearance of the same patient after cleansing. No more than light dressing was required after this step.

3 Appearance of a young man after a motor-cycle accident.

4 Appearance of the same patient after cleansing; the white streaks are burns caused by contact with the hot cylinder block. Their depth was not certain so they were allowed to heal. Six months later they had formed hypertrophic scars, which were later reduced by surgical abrasion and natural shrinkage.

Comment It can be helpful to be able to give the patient, especially a female one, some idea early on about the course of events and likely final cosmetic appearance.

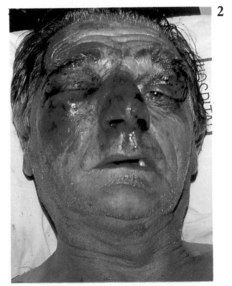

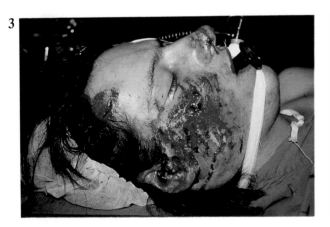

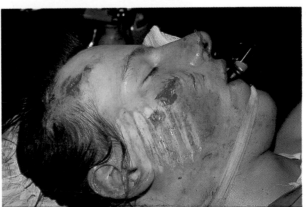

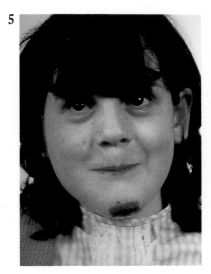

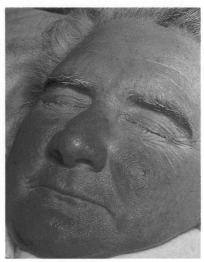

5 A graze or wound caused by a fall on to the point of the chin may be accompanied by damage to the incisor teeth, the neck(s) of the mandible or the anterior wall of the external auditory meatus, which can cause bleeding from the earhole.

6 The graze in the hair-line was made when this woman's brow struck the rim of a windscreen of a car that was in collision with another. She was conscious and complained of discomfort in the neck. (A collar can just be made out.) In spite of the appparent triviality of the graze, the force of the blow was sufficient to cause fractures of the arch of C1 and the body of C2.

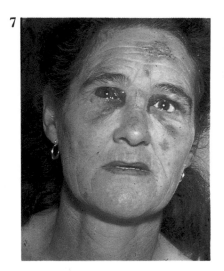

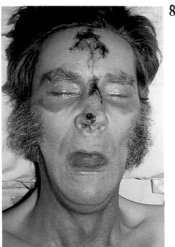

7 Bruising caused by a husband's punch. This woman attended hospital only because the police advised her to. When about to leave she mentioned discomfort on her neck. Xrays showed a fracture of the body of C6.

Comment Even the slightest mark of injury of the face or brow may be the sign of a blow that carried sufficient force to break the neck. Beyond middle-age, the neck is particularly vulnerable to sudden hyperextension, which can cause paralysis even though there is no fracture.

8 Injuries caused by a fall downstairs after drinking alcohol. The man had not been unconscious and was allowed to go home after being given local analgesia and having his wounds stitched. The following morning he returned because his neck was stiff and uncomfortable. Xrays showed a fracture of the odontoid process of the axis.

9 This man fell at work and knocked himself out. When he regained consciousness a few seconds later, he had to call for help to get up. His hands were paralysed by a lower motor neurone lesion and his lower limbs were weakened by an upper motor neurone lesion. There was well-marked cervical spondylosis but no fracture.

Comment Acute traumatic, spondylotic, cervical myelopathy occurs when the spinal cord is compressed between the permanent intervertebral bulge in front and the forward bulging of posterior soft tissues that takes place during forcible extension of the neck. It is a tragic consequence of an apparently mild injury and condemns the victim to permanent paralysis of the hands, although the lower limbs recover well. In this case the story, the mark on the brow and the age of the patient were typical of the condition, which was not diagnosed initially.

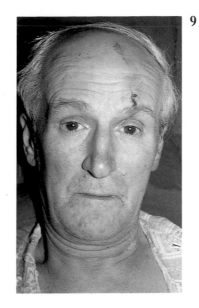

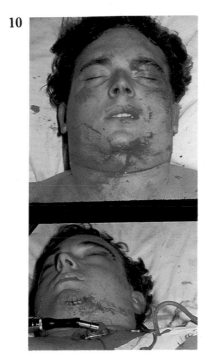

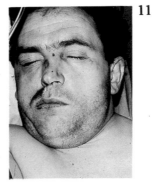

11 This man was reported to have banged his head when he walked into a bus, which he had dented. The time and day of the accident and his condition on admission suggested that the man was drunk. However, at the time that this photograph was taken, the small area of surgical emphysema that had been found low down at the back of his chest by an alert and painstaking senior house surgeon, had spread widely and caused the marked swelling of the neck and face.

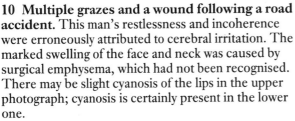

10 Multiple grazes and a wound following a road accident. This man's restlessness and incoherence were erroneously attributed to cerebral irritation. The marked swelling of the face and neck was caused by surgical emphysema, which had not been recognised. There may be slight cyanosis of the lips in the upper photograph; cyanosis is certainly present in the lower one.

Comment Both these men had clear evidence of injury of the head, and their behaviour was at first thought to be explicable by this. In fact, both had sustained serious injuries of the chest and were showing signs of cerebral hypoxia, which should be suspected when marked restlessness and even aggressive behaviour occur without provocation. When there has been physical damage to the brain, violent behaviour is unusual and when it does occur such behaviour is usually in response to being disturbed. In brief, the hypoxic patient goes for you whereas the victim of cerebral contusion tries to get away from you.

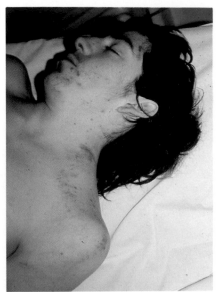

12 Although they were small, the grazes on the left side of the head and the shoulder suggested that the two had been forced apart, as by a fall or a road accident. The swelling in the supraclavicular fossa added to the suspicion that the upper part of the brachial plexus might have been injured in this unconscious man. A traction lesion was confirmed when he regained consciousness (*see* also **428**).

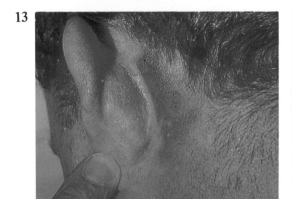

13 A bruise that had tracked down from a fracture.

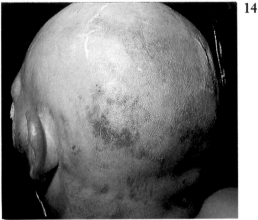

14 This mark was hidden until the hair had been removed. It overlay a fracture. A bruise of the scalp sometimes denotes the site of an extradural haemorrhage.

The eye

Any damage near the eye may be accompanied by damage to the eye itself. Examination can be hampered considerably by swelling and may have to be carried out under local anaesthesia.

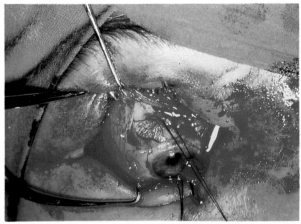

15 Obvious damage to the cornea was present but it was accompanied by damage to the conjunctiva further back.

Wounds

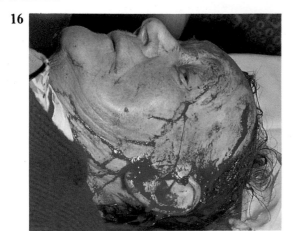

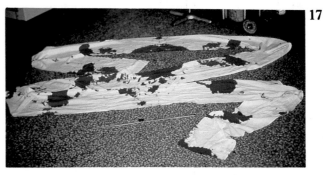

16 Even small wounds of the scalp can bleed profusely. Firm, local pressure will usually stop the bleeding. Close inspection identifies the large amount of blood in this old woman's hair. Dressings and clothing may also be soaked and the patient may collapse from loss of blood, which can continue profusely while stitches are being inserted but be hidden under a towel.

17 The amount of dressing is less important than the accurate placing of pressure; some 15 feet of roller towel did little to stop the bleeding from a 1½ inch cut on the back of the head. Sometimes both ends of a spurting artery need to be clipped.

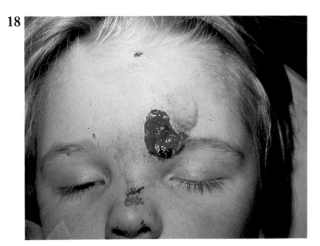

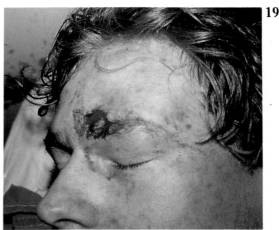

18 A small wound caused by a blow; the suspected underlying fracture was more easily identified by the naked eye during exploration than on xray films.

19 This similar looking wound was caused by a dog-bite; there was no loss of tissue and it was easily sewn up after trimming.

20 Even a narrow stalk of lip can sustain a flap like this one. There was no loss of tissue and it was sewn up. It requires great care to avoid irregularity of the red margin and the edge of the lip.

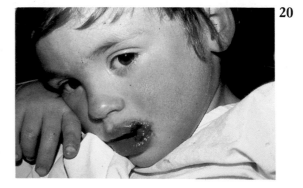

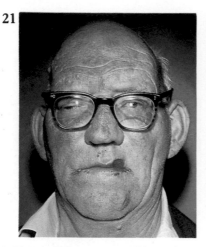

21

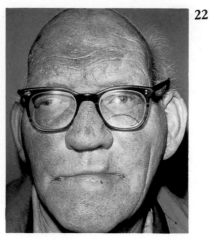

22

21 Superficial loss of tissue caused by a dog-bite.

22 V-excision gave a satisfactory cosmetic appearance 8 months later and perhaps looks better than a skin graft would have done.

23

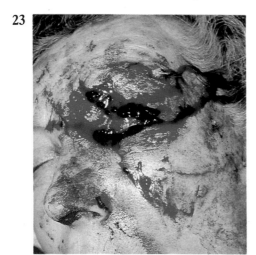

23 In spite of its threatening appearance, this wound spared the eyeball. When the lids are screwed up in reaction to a threat, there may be nearly half an inch of tissue in front of the eyeball.

24 This man had been stabbed in the left cheek some days before. A healing wound was present in the tongue and the slight swelling below the jaw on the right suggested that the knife had penetrated that far.

25 In spite of its site and severity, this large flap wound did no damage to the parotid gland, its duct or the facial nerve.

24

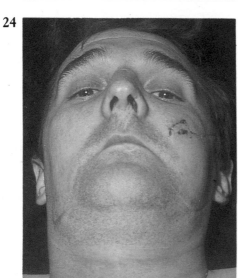

25

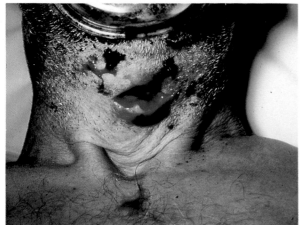

26 A self-inflicted stab wound that was more than 12 hours old and had entered the pharynx.

Comment Both deliberate and accidental stab wounds can be unexpectedly deep and they require careful exploration.

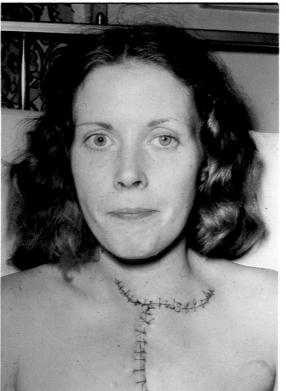

27 The incision shown was used to deal with a stab wound just above the clavicle that had divided the common carotid artery and the sympathetic chain. Note the drooping left eyelid and small left pupil.

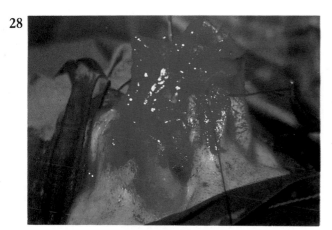

28 Wound of nose. Given the necessary skill, materials and patience, even complicated wounds can heal very well.

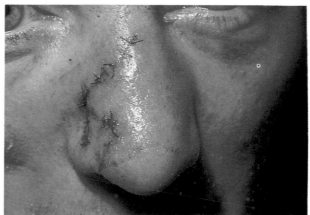

29 Time spent on proper care at the first operation is never wasted.

Comment When the full thickness of a muscular part has been injured, it must be repaired in layers if twitching scars are to be avoided.

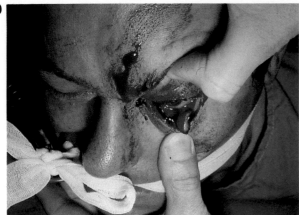

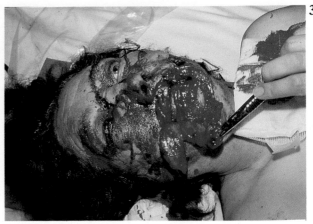

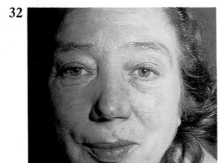

30 A wound near the medial canthus of the eyelid may cut the lacrimal duct. Particularly in the lower eyelid, this must be looked for and repaired if necessary.

31 The lips had been sliced through and have been turned back.

32 The resting posture of the same face a year later. Movements of the mouth and lips had recovered remarkably well.

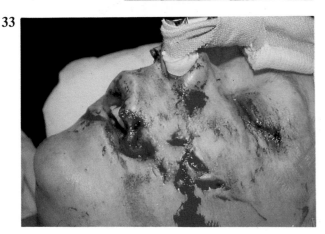

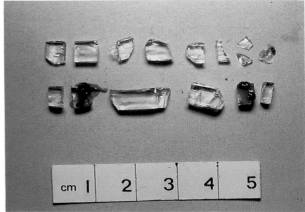

33 Wounds caused by broken glass thrown from a shattered car windscreen may not look very serious, but they can penetrate deeply and do a great deal of damage.

34 Glass fragments. After the initial operation, it is wise to warn the victim that some fragments of glass may have not been found. The dissection of too thorough a search can add considerably to the damage, whereas any remaining glass that later gives rise to complaint can usually be removed without difficulty. A written statement to this effect and signed by the patient is a valuable part of the notes.

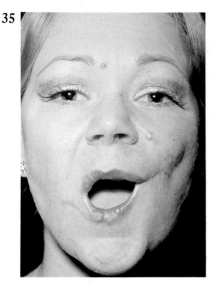

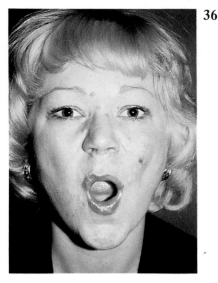

35 **In this case there was mild infection** with considerable scarring after three weeks.

36 **The same patient's cosmetic appearance after about a year was satisfactory.**

Comment Any request for plastic surgery should be resisted for about a year. Sound advice about the use of make-up in the meantime can help a distressed or impatient woman to be patient. In the end it may turn out to be that this is all that is required.

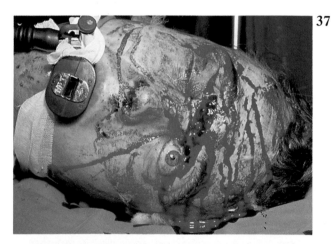

37 **The prominence of the left eye was caused by fragments of glass from a broken windscreen** that entered the orbit above the eyeball. On admission the eye could register only movements of a hand. However, good vision was restored a few weeks after the prompt removal of the glass allowed the eye to return to its rightful place.

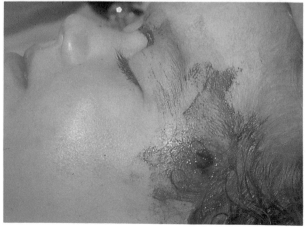

Gunshot wounds
38 **The powder marks show that this wound was inflicted at close range;** the 0.22 inch bullet came to rest near the pituitary fossa. Apart from mild and temporary paresis of the oculomotor nerve, there was no neurological damage. The bullet was not removed and the child made a complete recovery.

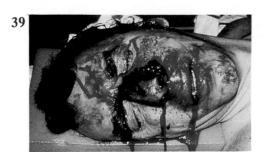

39 Attempted suicide by placing the muzzle of a shotgun in the mouth. As often happens during such attempts, the muzzle slipped as the trigger was pulled and the damage, although severe, was largely confined to the nose. In spite of the destructive nature of such a wound, primary closure may be possible. In the face, primary closure of untidy gunshot wounds is permissible, although infection will occur if surgical toilet is inadequate. It is wise to seek expert advice as soon as possible after this sort of injury.

Exploration of wounds and foreign bodies

This topic deserves careful consideration because many so-called minor wounds are dealt with by junior doctors that have had no detailed instruction on how to go about it; as a result they may do no good and, even worse, cause much damage. General consideration will be given now and particular points will be emphasised as appropriate in later chapters.

The purpose is to reveal the full depth and extent of the damage and allow dead tissue and foreign matter to be found and removed. Sometimes the combination of reassuring xray appearances and clinical signs makes it unnecessary to explore a wound; for example the case shown in **38**.

Exploration

1 A probe, or a finger if the wound is large enough, can give a useful indication of the direction of a wound but neither is a reliable guide to depth.

2 A wound that penetrates several layers or structures may seem much shallower than it is, because an alteration of posture from that at the time of injury can break up the track as the layers move on each other.

3 Not all wounds need to be enlarged; the careful use of retractors and fine instruments may reveal all that needs to be seen.

4 When extension of a wound is necessary, it should give comfortable access and it should be made with due regard to the direction of the wound, the tissues at risk and its possible effect on the viability of the skin; its relationship to creases and the risk of hypertrophic scarring are of secondary importance at this stage.

5 When a tendon is seen in a wound, it should be watched throughout its excursion in case damage to it has moved out of sight.

6 Dissection should be kept to a minimum while injured structures are being identified; dissection disturbs natural relationships and can thereby greatly increase the difficulties of identification. There is no shame in consulting a textbook of anatomy during an operation.

7 A tourniquet is a valuable aid to exploration of a limb, otherwise the part should be kept as high as possible in relation to the rest of the body. Irrigation and suction may also help.

Foreign bodies

1 Not all need to be removed.

2 A possible foreign body that cannot be identified on xray films (for example, fabric, wood or a plastic material) should not necessarily be sought surgically, because this can do a great deal of damage and no good.

3 If a foreign body is present and not already visible in the wound, the following precautions should be taken.

4 Regard the operation as difficult until it has been successfully completed.

5 Use a form of anaesthesia that can be prolonged for as long as necessary.

6 Have a bloodless field whenever possible.

7 Have a good light and an assistant available if needed.

8 Have xray films of the part in the position in which it is to be operated on.

9 Try to work out the layer(s) in which the foreign body lies. Sharp objects such as needles are often stopped by bone and may be in contact with it.

10 Needles should not be approached down their tracks (which are usually unrecognisable) but across their length; like ships, they are easier targets from abeam than from astern. These rules are more easily stated than followed, except by those who have been taught properly or have learned their lesson the hard way, that is at the patients' expense. Most failures occur because the surgeon sets out confidently and single-handed and uses local infiltration analgesia.

Ingrained dirt

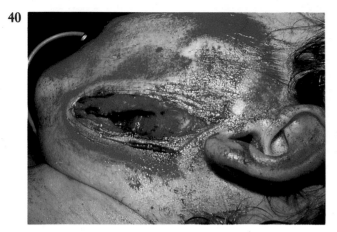

40 Ingrained dirt should be removed when the wound is first treated. Scraping with the point of a fine knife is more precise than scrubbing with a brush and may be more effective. The abrasions in front of the ear were dealt with in this way. The dirty part of the wound that exposed the mandible was cut out and the wound was stitched.

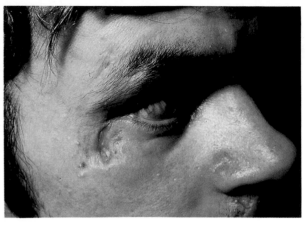

41 The result of inadequate primary treatment of a dirty, gouged wound.

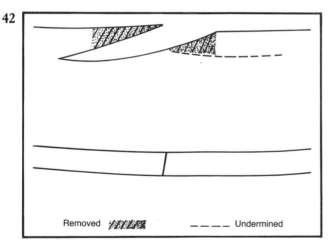

Removed ▨▨▨▨   – – – – Undermined

42 Slicing flap wounds should be trimmed to create square edges, which are then advanced.

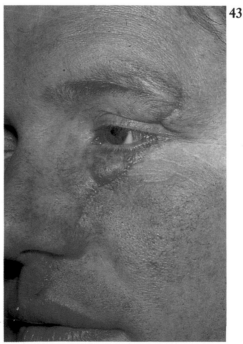

43 Even so, the lower edge of the flap may show dependent oedema for some months, during which firm massage may be helpful. When tissue has been lost, ugly deformity can result but all too often this sort of appearance is the result of inadequate care.

Wounds of the brain

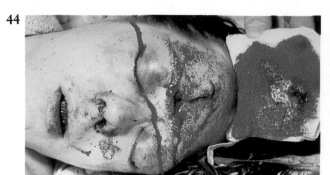

44

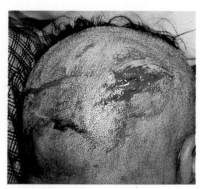

45

44 The fact that some wounds have damaged the skull and even the brain may be obvious. Some brain is visible on the swab but this man made a good recovery in all respects.

45 A blow by a hard object that does not cause unconsciousness may appear to have damaged the scalp only, but the skull must be xrayed and the wound must be explored.

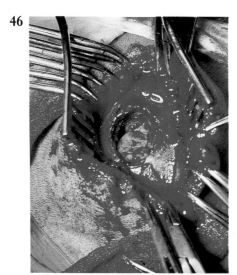

46

46 A fracture that is known to be open and depressed must be explored because foreign matter, particularly hair, is often trapped in it.

The ear

47 A partly detached pinna should be stitched back without delay. This one healed perfectly. Complete or nearly complete detachment is irreparable; the defect should be grafted and may be hidden by the hair, which should not be removed in preparation.

48 Loss of the rim can be treated with a split skin graft, if there is little or no bare cartilage. Exposed cartilage can be buried in the scalp. For some victims, this may be permanently satisfactory.

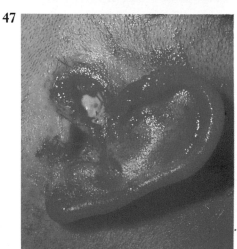

47

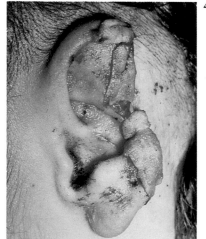

48

Swelling and deformity

49 Tensely swollen eyelids (note the swelling of the cheek, which has distorted the mouth) may prevent examination of the eye. Leeches (perhaps 3 or 4) can make it possible to part the lids. Biting is facilitated by placing a drop of sugared water on the lid. When sated, the leech will drop off. Although it will vomit if placed in salt water it may not regain its appetite for some time.

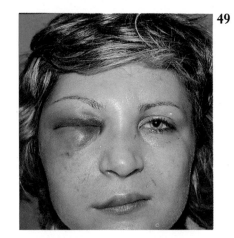

50 This girl was struck in the face. What seemed to be a mild bruise felt soft and crackly and was easily dented. A tangential xray view showed surgical emphysema but not the crack that had presumably breached the frontal sinus.

Fracture of the zygomatic bone

51 The wound of the brow and the subconjunctival haemorrhage were obvious, but there was also a mark over the cheekbone and swelling lower down.

52 Careful comparison of the two cheeks confirmed that there was depression of the body of the right zygomatic bone.

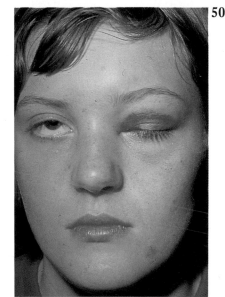

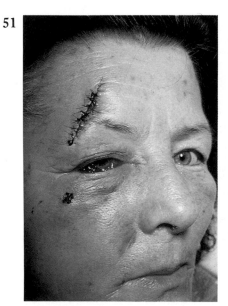

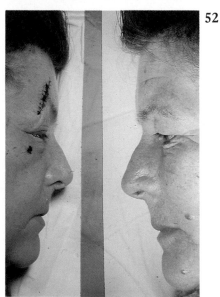

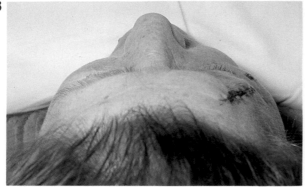

53 The usefulness of the supraorbital ridges for reference can be improved if one places the tips of one's straight forefingers on corresponding bony prominences in the cheeks. There may also be bleeding from the nostril, numbness of the cheek and upper lip and incisor teeth on the affected side. Very rarely the eye is blind; vision must be tested before any corrective operation is undertaken.

Comment The inexperienced emergency room officer tends to place too much reliance on xray films, which can be confusing, and not enough on the careful systematic clinical examination of the injured person.

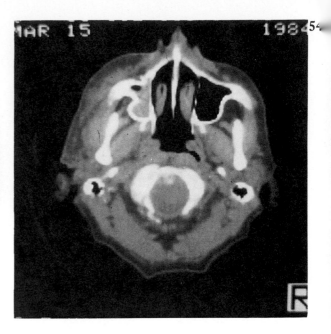

54 Use of CT. Where it is available, computed tomography shows the displacement of fragments very clearly.

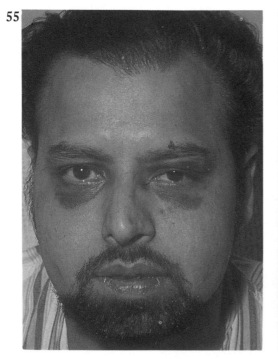

55 This man was punched in the face. Although he had more bruising on the right than on the left, the left cheek looked slightly more swollen; it also crackled because of surgical emphysema.

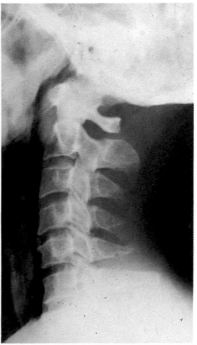

56 The surgical emphysema spread to the prevertebral plane. Presumably there had been a fracture into the maxillary sinus and air had tracked from there.

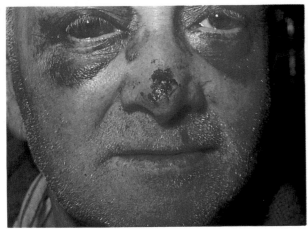

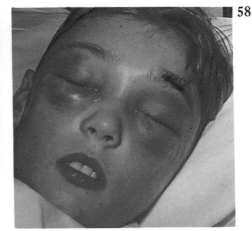

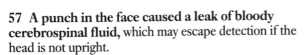

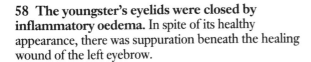

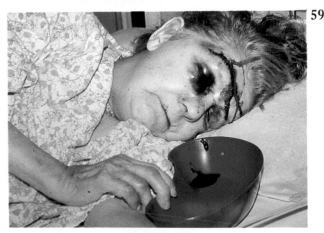

57 A punch in the face caused a leak of bloody cerebrospinal fluid, which may escape detection if the head is not upright.

58 The youngster's eyelids were closed by inflammatory oedema. In spite of its healthy appearance, there was suppuration beneath the healing wound of the left eyebrow.

59 Two black eyes, bleeding from the nose and unconsciousness make the recovery position an obvious choice. Unfortunately, this old woman had a broken odontoid process. Unless the recovery position is adopted very carefully and no less carefully maintained, it can endanger the spinal cord.

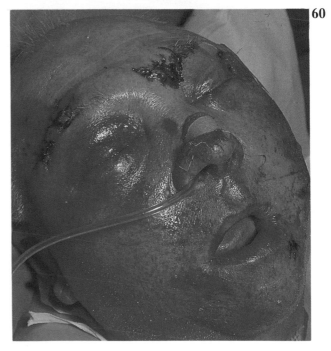

60 The typical football face with a button nose that developed after a fracture of the middle third of the face and hid the bony deformity.

Comment There was no fracture in the neck. Such patients are in danger of choking to death, because of both bleeding into the pharynx and its blockage by swollen and displaced tissues. Intubation may be urgently necessary but extremely difficult especially if the victim is partly conscious or very restless. It is a procedure that requires great skill.

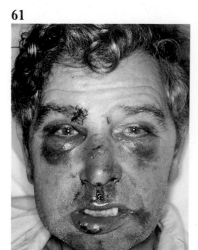

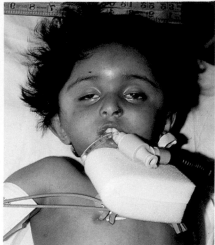

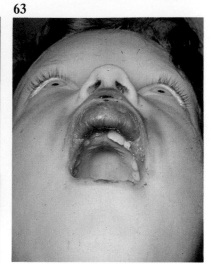

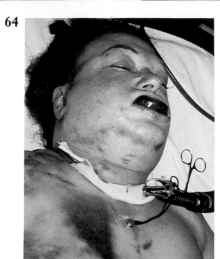

64

61 The appearance of a dish-face before swelling had obscured the flattening.

62 Massive swelling beneath the scalp after an extensive fracture.

63 Ugly but localised and harmless swelling of the upper lip that had almost disappeared after a week. The teeth were undamaged.

64 Massive and extensive swelling of the chest and neck and within the mouth that required tracheostomy. The dark red band beneath the nose was sublingual haematoma that had protruded from the mouth.

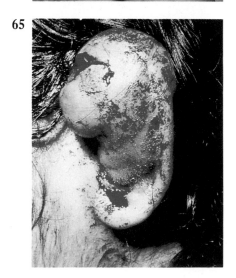

65

65 A thick ear, more formally known as a haematoma of the pinna. Even prompt decompression, which requires generous incision, not aspiration, did not completely prevent the cauliflower ear that results from death of the cartilage.

66 The rapid and severe swelling of the eyelids and profuse bleeding from the nose and mouth betokened a very severe injury. The patient died shortly afterwards.

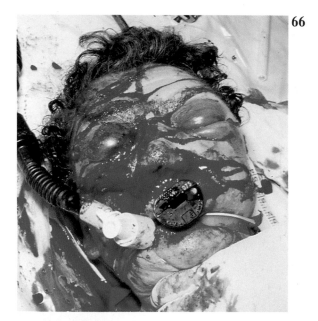

66

67 and **68 Severe fracture of the base of the skull.** If still alive when they reach hospital, patients with brain coming from the nose, mouth or ear, (it can be seen on the dressing below) especially if there is also profuse bleeding from the mouth, have severe and extensive fractures of the base of the skull (**68**). Such victims should not be given priority over others with a chance of surviving.

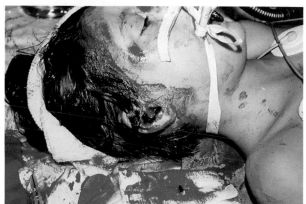

67

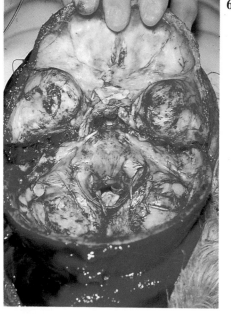

68

Other conditions

Posture

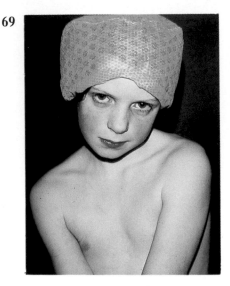

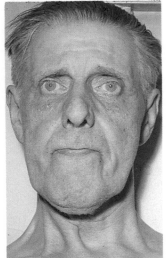

69 This child was not being coy; she had acute wry neck, which may or may not have a recognisable cause such as a wrench, blow or unusual action.

70 The slight asymmetry of the face and neck was the result of a broken odontoid process that caused little discomfort.

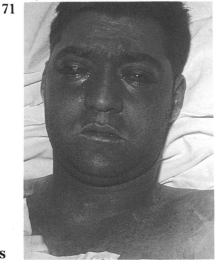

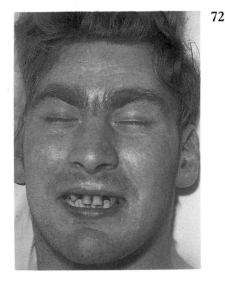

Expressions

71 The discoloration of traumatic asphyxia, which results from relatively slow but forcible compression of the chest. Even the light pressure of clothing can be enough to prevent the change of colour. There may be no fractures and little difficulty in breathing; the condition is usually more frightening than serious.

Prolapse of the conjunctiva caused in this way soon goes down, unlike that associated with massive, tense swelling, which is capable of causing strangulation and sloughing.

72 Mild tetanus. This man's mouth could not be opened any more widely than shown as a result of the onset of mild tetanus about 10 days after a wound of the leg that looked healthy. The man recovered.

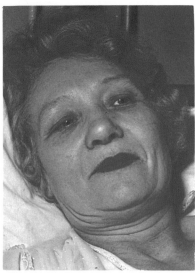
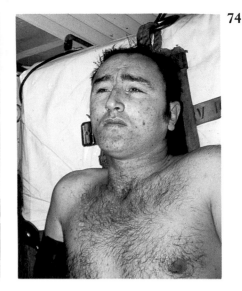

73 An expression of quiet challenge that accompanied complaints for which no physical explanation could be found.

74 This man was reported to have been paralysed after a fall. He was admirably splinted on the way to hospital by means of a Neil-Robertson stretcher. The tense set of his face and narrowed eyelids, which showed a fine tremor, was striking. He made a rapid recovery from the effects of his fright.

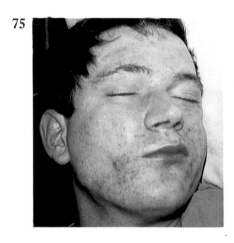
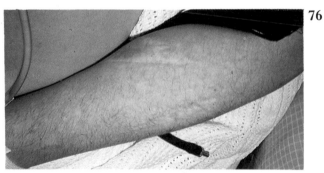

75 This youth was found collapsed and apparently unrousable outside the front entrance of the Birmingham Accident Hospital not very late one New Year's Eve. His face was not devoid of expression. Sometimes one sees fine tremor or even blinking movements of the closed eyelids; these are not features of coma.

76 These were fine linear scars on the fronts of the left forearm and also the shoulder and wrist, where a right-handed person might cut himself. The youth remained in his apparently unrousable state until he was ready to go home the next morning, when he dressed and left.

3 The trunk

Although the chest and belly are anatomically distinct and separate parts of the trunk, as far as injury is concerned, they cannot always be considered separately.

It is perhaps with injuries of the chest that a discerning eye can provide more useful information than with injuries anywhere else in the body. The evidence available includes:

- Respiratory distress
- Cyanosis, which may be masked by blood, dirt, poor light or dark skin
- Venous congestion
- Bruises, grazes and wounds
- Swelling
- Asymmetry of shape and movement of chest

Taken in conjunction with other means of clinical examination, visible signs will often at least arouse suspicion and sometimes they leave no doubt about the diagnosis. A particular example is a rapidly expanding pneumothorax that requires immediate venting. Waiting for xray films may be fatal when there are obvious signs of respiratory distress, venous congestion and cyanosis of the head and neck, prominence of one side of the chest with little or no movement on breathing, absent or much reduced breath sounds therein, and displacement of the trachea and apex beat of the heart.

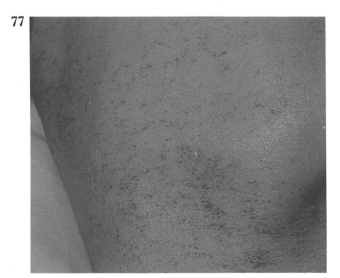

77

77 Fat embolism. This is often equated with a few scattered petechiae in the region of the shoulders. However, it can affect the chest lower down and the spots are sometimes numerous, as appeared over this man's right costal margin.

Comment The presence or absence of spots is of little practical importance. The syndrome attributed to fat embolism is most likely after fractures of long bones and, most of all, the pelvis. The careful observer will not overlook slight cyanosis, an anxious expression, slightly increased rate and depth of respiration, which may be accompanied by mild fever, confusion and restlessness, and incontinence of urine. Although profuse petechial haemorrhages may be found in the brain post mortem, complete recovery can follow coma, even with focal neurological signs.

Bruises and grazes

78 This man was struck in the chest by the steering wheel of a car that crashed. The marks of impact were visible, if not very striking. It should be noted that although the lips were of normal colour, the man's neck was cyanotic and the external jugular vein was prominent. The combination suggested that there was local venous obstruction caused by, for example, mediastinal haematoma, possibly owing to rupture of the aorta, pericardial tamponade or contusion of the myocardium. Further evidence supported the last. The bulges at the base of the neck were made by the normal clavicles.

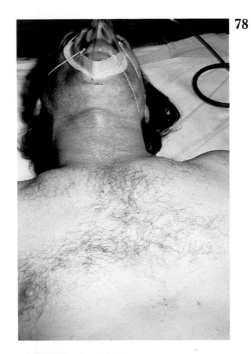

79 The graze behind the lower part of the chest was obvious; less obvious was the mark towards the front and higher up. The two marks were caused by crushing and the resulting distortion of the chest ruptured the diaphragm and bisected the spleen. He survived.

Comment(i) The surgeon must decide whether to explore through the chest or the abdomen; either approach can be extended but, when abdominal viscera may have been injured, the abdominal approach usually suffices with left-sided injuries. (ii) Although the ribs often protect the viscera from forces that do obvious damage to the skin, do not assume this without good reason.

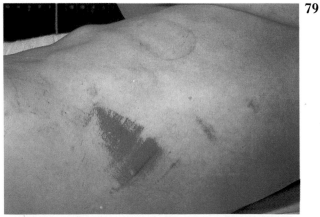

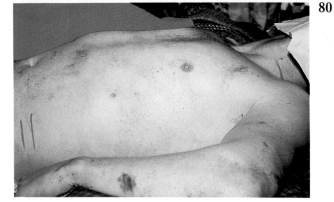

80 Marks of impact sustained by the front-seat passenger in a car crash.

81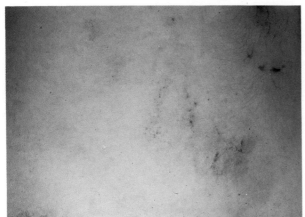

81 Same patient as in 80. Close inspection identified purplish-brown spotty bruising below the left ribs as well as the mild grazes on the chest. Spotty bruising on skin that does not have bone close beneath it is strong evidence of damage to abdominal viscera. In this case the spleen was ruptured. The fact that the left arm was broken, presumably while it was against his side, provided strong evidence of the force of impact on the casualty's trunk.

82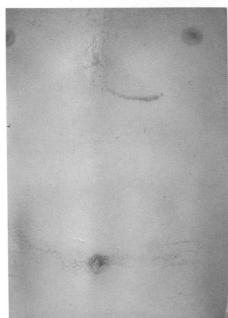

82 A well-marked band of spotty bruising that was caused by a steering wheel that had been dented by the impact and had crushed the jejunum and greater omentum against the spine.

83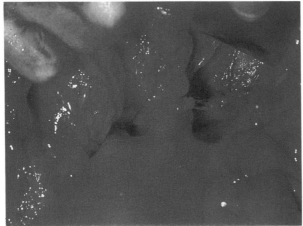

83 Spotty bruising. In another case, impact by a steering wheel caused similar spotty bruising and transected the right rectus abdominis, partly transected the left and caused numerous bruises and splits affecting the gut and the peritoneum in both iliac fossae. The pinkish-golden triangle adjoining the retractor at 2 o'clock is the left anterior sacroiliac ligament, which had been exposed by the injury; the overlying soft tissues had been crushed through.

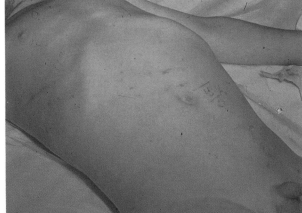

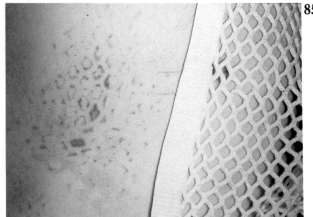

84 Fractured pelvis. This boy was in coma and had a clinically obvious fracture of the pelvis after being knocked down in the road. On close inspection, the faint marks below the left ribs were seen to be spotty bruises. Had peritoneal lavage been in use in 1966, it would have been positive and might have been attributed, like his pallor, to the fracture of the pelvis. Because of the marks the belly was explored; there was a rupture of the spleen and there were two tears in the mesentery of the small intestine. He later died of his cerebral injury.

85 The term 'pattern bruising' has been used to describe these marks but the words are better reserved for cases in which bruising has a definite pattern. On close inspection of the bruising on this man's belly, it could be seen that the bruising occurred immediately adjacent to the strings of the vest and not under them; in this respect it had something in common with traumatic asphyxia (71), in that it was the result of relatively gentle pressure and was therefore unlikely to denote internal injury; such was this case.

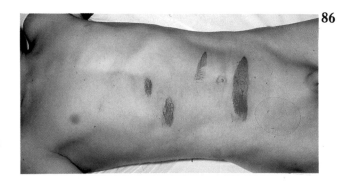

86 The history suggested that these were friction burns and the appearance of the boy's vest confirmed it. Internal injury is not likely in these circumstances and was not present in this case.

Comment Spotty bruising of skin that is close to bone has something in common with the striking of a coin or a medal and it may have a fracture under it. When spotty bruising appears on skin without immediate bony support, it means that the skin has been driven hard against bone and that in most cases there has been noteworthy damage to the intervening structures. Unless such damage can be ruled out by other investigations, this sign calls for laparotomy. Its importance is such that it should be looked for deliberately. If nurses see spotty bruising when they are undressing a patient, they should report it to a doctor immediately.

Wounds

Stabbing is now the most frequent cause of penetrating wounds of the chest in the UK, but it occurs much less frequently than in some other countries. Because stab wounds are often multiple, the patient must be examined carefully all the way round.

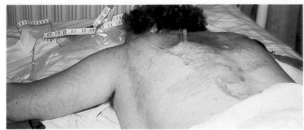

87 A stab in the back. In this case the clinical and radiological evidence made it clear that there was no need for exploration.

Comment Penetrating wounds below the nipple and in the front or side of the chest may have entered the abdominal cavity. With such wounds, free gas or blood in the peritoneal cavity suggests that exploration should be considered, if only because stab wounds of the diaphragm can be followed years later by herniation and strangulation of gut.

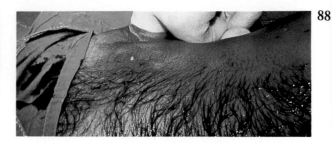

88 Stab wound in the flank. Although it was obviously more than skin deep, a probing finger found that this stab wound went upwards and was above the diaphragm. On the operating table, and under general anaesthesia, the finger is a legitimate and sometimes very useful guide to the direction, if not the depth, of a wound.

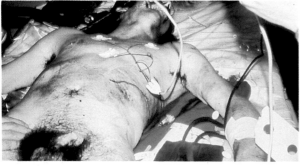

89 Stab wounds of the heart may require immediate and massive intravenous infusion through several cannulae, prompt thoracotomy (in the emergency room), cross-clamping of the aorta above the diaphragm, and temporary occlusion of one or more holes in the heart or great vessels. Definitive repair would then be carried out in a fully equipped operating theatre. Given these facilities, American experience suggests that 10-15 per cent of such cases may be saved, although in some instances signs of life ceased before the victim reached hospital.

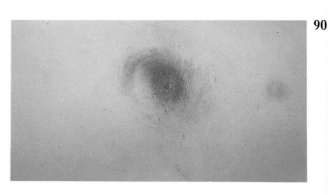

90 The powder marks of a gunshot wound below the nipple and at close range. Relatively slow missiles such as a 0.22 inch bullet may not follow a direct line from the point of entry to the point of lodgement, which was behind the heart and near the spine. Because there was no sign of damage to important structures, no operation was carried out. The child remained well and retained the bullet (*see* also **38**).

91 A large wound caused by an industrial accident. The lung was visible through the wound and had been re-expanded by artificial ventilation. If the lung is airtight, this is a better aid to breathing than merely sealing the wound. In any case, an air drain should be placed in the chest. In spite of appearances, no tissue had been lost and simple toilet and suture were all that was required.

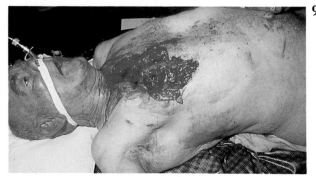

91

Selective exploration of stab wounds

Although American and South African reports have shown that about 50 per cent of stab wounds of the belly do little or no internal damage and that the decision whether or not to explore can usually be based on careful and repeated clinical examination, some surgeons in these and other countries prefer to explore every case, although negative exploration is not without its complications. Peritoneal lavage is more reliable than might be supposed, but whether or not the wound can be shown to enter the peritoneal cavity cannot be relied upon for deciding for or against exploration.

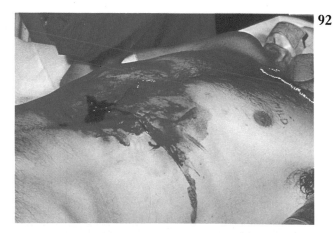

92

92 A stab wound that had caused profuse bleeding and obviously needed to be explored. It was found that the knife had pierced the liver, the lesser omentum, the pancreas and had entered the splenic vein. The man recovered.

93 A loop of gut that emerged through a stab wound. The same can happen with a gunshot wound; in either case the belly must be explored.

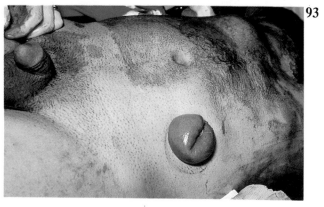

93

Comment Stabbing often occurs after the victim has had a good deal to eat and drink, especially alcohol. A stomach tube needs to be passed, but, as in this case, it should not be done until blood is running into the patient. If this precaution is not taken, the disturbance of passing the tube may set off profuse bleeding and endanger the victim's life.

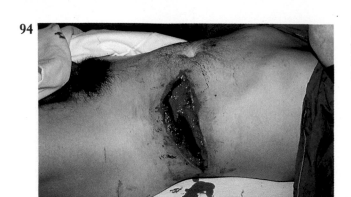

94 This large wound was caused when a powered saw broke. Xrays and exploration confined to the wound showed that laparotomy was not necessary.

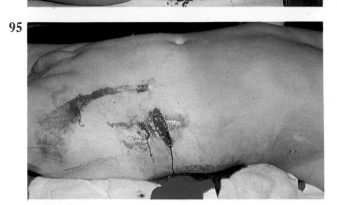

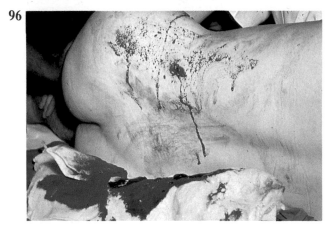

95 and **96 The man shown was struck above the left iliac crest by a heavy coil of wire as it fell.** The two small wounds and the graze did not look serious but the skin over the upper part of the sacrum appeared to be bulging and there had been appreciable external bleeding; the man was also pale. On joining the wounds it was obvious that the muscles of the flank had been stripped from the iliac crest.

97 and 98 The blue line showed the extent of undermining of the skin that was found during the operation. The man made a good recovery.

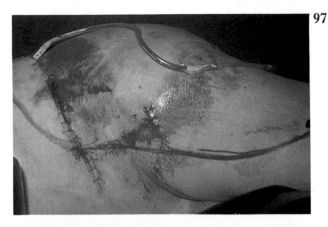

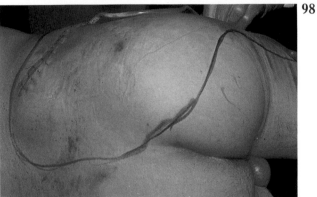

99 Transfixion may do remarkably little internal damage if the transfixing agent is blunt but this splinter of wood, which entered the right side of the chest, carried in and jammed clothing around it, pierced the diaphragm and tore the spleen, stomach and liver. This man made a good recovery.

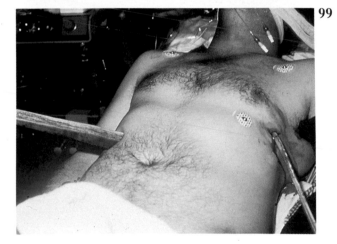

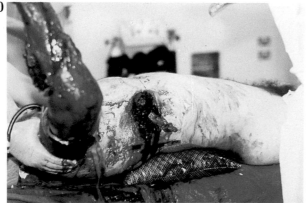

100 This impalement injury occurred when a car collided with metal railings at high speed. Pulped liver was visible beneath the broken rib.

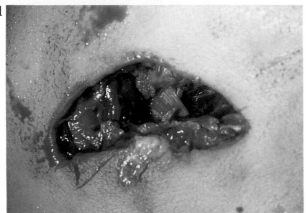

101 On the back of the same victim was another wound. It communicated with the first and on careful examination the dura mater could be seen (bluish, near the top edge of the wound) where part of the neural arch had been carried away. The man died on the operating table.

Swelling and deformity

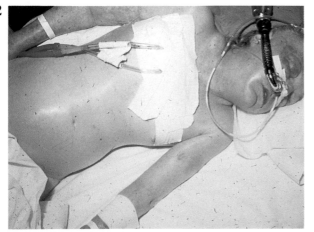

102 Marked swelling caused by surgical emphysema that had reached the full extent that is anatomically possible—from the eyebrows to the groins, where at the plane of cleavage is closed by the fusion of the two layers of the superficial fascia. The drainage tubes (one should be enough) led into the pleural cavity.

Comment Even light pressure indents this sort of swelling, which fills out again after a few seconds. The place where surgical emphysema first appears is of diagnostic value. If it begins at the root of the neck, it usually means that the air has come from the trachea or a bronchus. Otherwise it comes from the lung.

103 The genitals of a man can be affected by surgical emphysema.

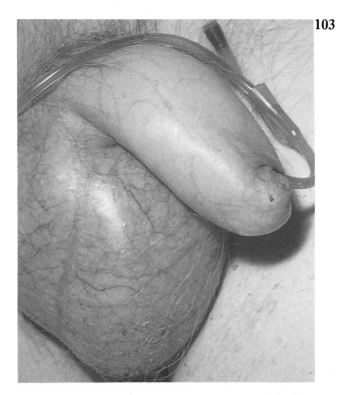

104 An unusual example of surgical emphysema that was still mild enough to produce a lumpy swelling rather than smooth distension.

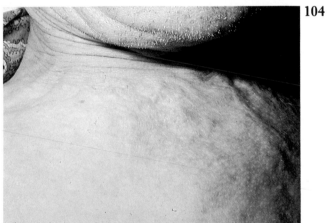

105 Asymmetry resulting mostly from bruising although a large, tense pneumothorax might have been responsible.

Comment When the chest is asymmetrical it is not always as obvious as in this case which is the injured side.

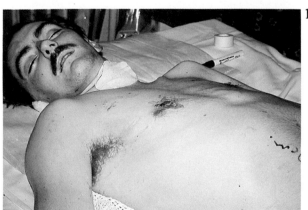

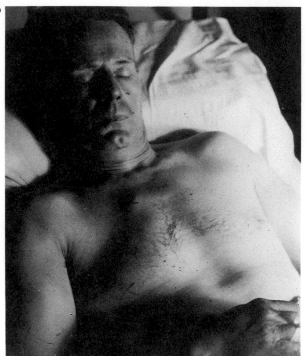

106 Asymmetry of shape after the chest had been crushed between railway buffers. When the man breathed there was obvious asymmetry of movement as well as of shape and the depressed area moved paradoxically.

Comment The flexible chests of children and young adults can show marked paradoxical movement as a result of rapid, deep breathing and without any fractures.

107

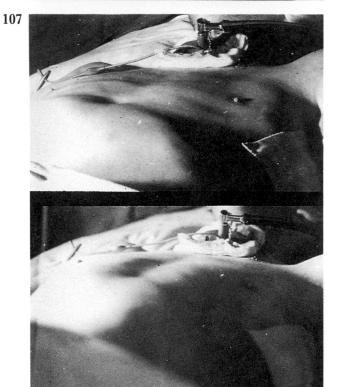

107 Inspiration and expiration after injury. The upper photograph was taken during inspiration and showed flattening of the left side of the chest when compared with the lower photograph, which was taken during expiration. This may be the result of multiple fractures of ribs but when an oral or nasal endotracheal tube is in place, paradoxical movement of the whole of the left side of the chest may be owing to the fact that the tube has been passed too far and has entered the right main bronchus and blocked the left. If this is the case, there is no sound of air passing in and out of the lung; natural movements and sounds are restored by pulling the tube out an inch or so. A tracheostomy tube is too short to act in this way.

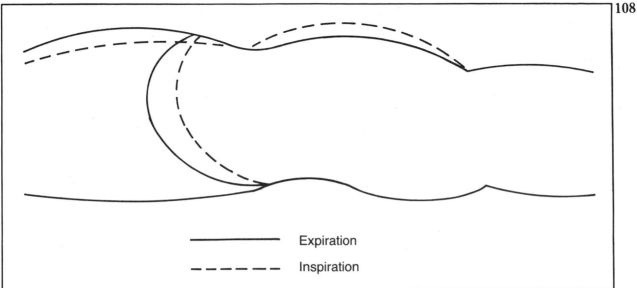

| Expiration |
| Inspiration |

108 Another sort of paradoxical movement is characterised by a see-saw movement of the chest and belly. The chest falls and the belly rises during inspiration and vice versa during expiration. This results from tetraplegia, when the diaphragm is the main active muscle of respiration. It can also occur during vigorous breathing by a person who normally uses mainly the diaphragm. Rarely, see-saw breathing occurs because multiple fractures of the back ends of ribs on both sides have virtually disconnected the rib cage from the spine and so deprived the intercostal muscles of their costovertebral fulcra.

Two further points about paradoxical movement of the chest need to be made.
1 At first it may be the only sign of serious injury because fractures, air and blood may not show in early xray films of the chest.
2 Paradoxical movement that comes on after a few hours is often the result of a complication such as collapse or diminished compliance of a lung. This is because it now requires more effort to breathe, which shows up instability of the chest wall that was not evident during gentler and slower breathing.

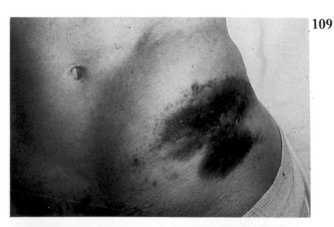

109 Fractures of the pelvis can cause massive swelling that can accommodate more than half the blood volume, but marked and more localised bruising such as this suggests that a large blood vessel has been injured; in this case it was the external iliac artery.

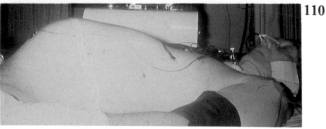

110 The prominence of this man's belly was the result of massive internal bleeding after a mild looking fracture of the pelvis. The source of the bleeding was the mesentery, not the pelvis or adjoining blood vessels. This is the sort of case in which angiography and therapeutic embolism might do away with the need for laparotomy.

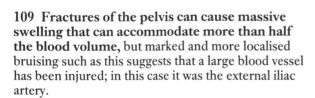

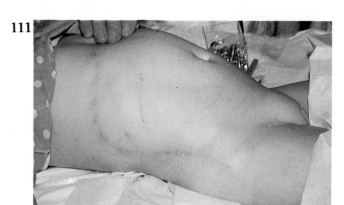

111 The curved bruise marks where this child was struck by a car. She was deathly pale and limp and had a distended belly. Resuscitation was attempted (note the fingers pressing on the sternum) but without success. There were severe ruptures of the liver and right kidney.

Comment The combination of exsanguination and limpness with a distended belly is of very grave significance. The heart stops because it is empty as a result of severe bleeding into the abdominal cavity.

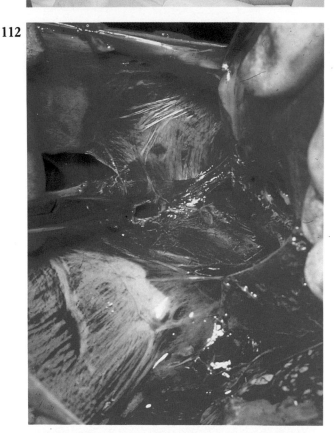

112 A child whose inferior vena cava had been torn across responded well to rapid infusion into tributaries of the superior vena cava but only slightly when tributaries of the inferior vena cava had to be used. When she relaxed under general anaesthesia her heart promptly stopped beating, because muscular tone no longer kept the two ends of the torn inferior vena cava together. One end can be seen on the under surface of the diaphragm. There was also rupture of the right suprarenal gland; as an isolated injury this would probably be of no importance to a survivor. The liver was almost uninjured.

Comment When there is evidence of severe bleeding into the belly, the upper limb(s) should be used for infusion in preference to the lower one(s).

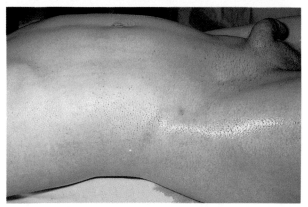

113 Tense swelling caused by a massive retroperitoneal haematoma from a shattered kidney. Note the increasingly obvious cyanosis below the waist that was the result of pressure on the inferior vena cava.

Peritoneal lavage

When there is reason to suspect injury in the belly, particularly in an unconscious person or other victim of multiple injuries, peritoneal lavage can be very helpful. The incision can be made after local anaesthesia has been induced. When the peritoneum has been exposed, all bleeding must be stopped before a dialysis catheter is pushed through it and down towards the pelvis. If there is not an immediate outflow of blood, 1 litre of saline is run in through the catheter and allowed to return by siphonage. There is no agreement about what constitutes a positive result sufficient to warrant laparotomy; opinions range from 20,000 to 100,000 red cells per mm^3.

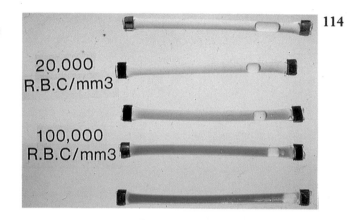

114

114 Red blood cells per mm^3. This chart shows the colours of dilutions from 10,000 to 150,000 red cells and enables the individual surgeon to decide in accordance with his own criteria whether or not to open the belly.

The back

No patient is too badly injured to be rolled carefully on to the side so that the back can be examined in detail, but a skilled team and adequate resuscitation are prerequisite. Be absolutely sure that the whole circumference of the patient has been examined thoroughly, lest stab wounds, for example, in the unexposed posterolateral strip escape detection.

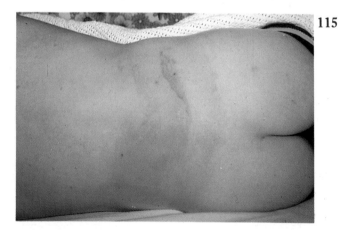

115

115 A van's wheel passed over the trunk of this person but there was no internal injury, probably because of the protective effect of the pelvis.

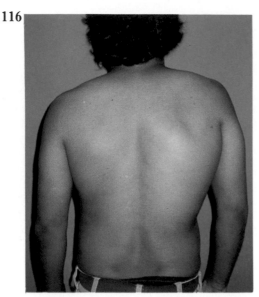

116 Extensive swelling that was the result of a large haematoma deep to latissimus dorsi that followed a kick during a game of rugby football. The swelling subsided without treatment.

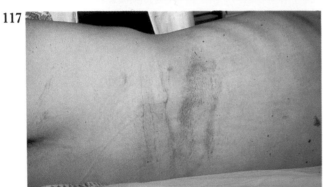

117 A bruise resulting from falling backwards across a beam. The associated hyperextension fracture of the pedicle did not prevent a rapid return to cautious activity.

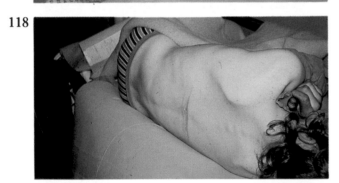

118 This transverse graze was caused by the edge of a tread when a youth fell down stairs. The lumbar curve had been reversed by a mild wedge fracture. There was little local swelling and no gap to feel.

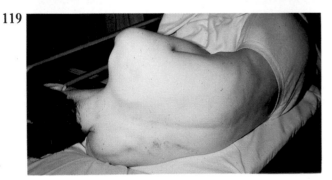

119 When a youth was flung out of a crashing vehicle, he landed on his shoulders. As well as the marks of impact, there was an accentuation of the thoracolumbar curve because of a wedge fracture. There was little local swelling and no gap to feel.

120 A heavy fall on to the back caused a fracture of T5 and T6 with paraplegia but little obvious swelling and no gap. The lesion was overlooked at the first hospital to which the victim was admitted.

Comment As well as looking at the back, one should run a finger firmly down the spinous processes and interspinous ligaments. A gap between two spinous processes is evidence of a disruptive injury that also tears the thoracolumbar fascia and causes obvious local bruising. The patients shown in **117-119** had mild fractures that did not endanger the spinal cord or its nerve roots.

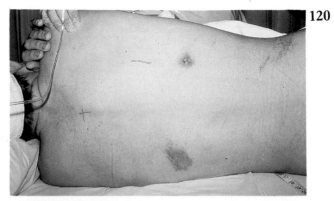

121 Fracture-dislocation with paraplegia. Here the gap between the spinous processes was much more obvious to the examiner's finger than to the observer's eye.

4 Shoulder to wrist

Bruises and grazes

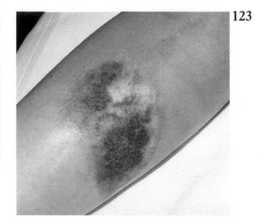

122 Spotty bruising on a well-padded part such as the shoulder signifies at least a fairly heavy blow but not usually a fracture. In a bulky shoulder it may not be easy to appreciate that these apparently unremarkable bruises are accompanied by extensive swelling, containing perhaps a litre or so of blood.

123 The appearance that can follow prolonged crushing such as occurs when an unconscious person lies on the part for some hours. At first, the site of pressure appears pale and sunken and because of the redness around it may be mistaken for a burn. If it is sufficiently severe and prolonged, the crushing also affects the muscles and nerves and results in at least temporary numbness and paralysis. Later, the ischaemic muscle may develop a contracture and should be excised.

Wounds

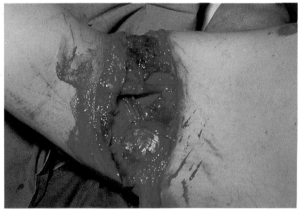

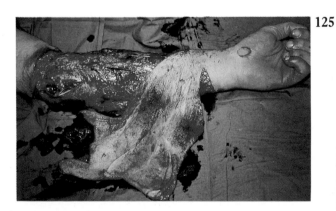

124 Although this wound in the axilla exposed the neurovascular bundle, the damage was confined to the skin, pectoralis major and latissimus dorsi and required no more than simple toilet and closure.

125 Extensive flaying caused when this limb was run over in the road. Damage is often confined to the skin but bones may be exposed.

126 In this case the elbow joint was opened and the articular surface of the trochlea of the humerus was just visible. Such severe damage to bone and joint is unusual and requires immediate internal fixation to prevent distortion of growth.

Comment Skin injured in this way does not survive and has usually been too badly damaged to be worth replacing after removing the fat, but it can be replaced by split skin grafts within 4 or 5 days.

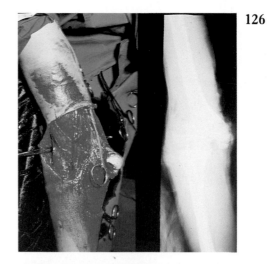

127 Extensive flaying and deeper damage of the entire forearm caused when a car rolled over on to a forearm that was resting on the edge of the open window. The bones were broken, the wound was 5 days old and it was superficially infected but the hand had an adequate circulation and nerve supply.

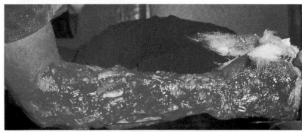

128 Four days after surgical toilet it was ready for split skin grafts. A nail was used in the radius to confer stability without an exposed implant (external fixation might be preferred now).

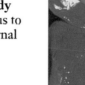

129 It may be worth replacing a skin flap a few inches across and securing it with stitches or, preferably, sticky strips, especially if it retains a proximal and reasonably broad base. In this case, the translucent appearance of the flap after about 10 days suggested that it had been quite badly crushed and would have been better removed at once. However, there was no sign of infection and the tissues beneath provided a good bed for split skin grafting.

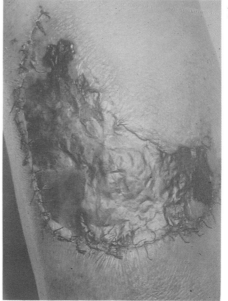

130 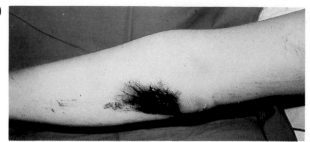 **A deep and dirty graze caused by a fall from a pedal cycle.** When there is skin to spare, it is simplest to cut out the dirty skin and sew up the rest.

131 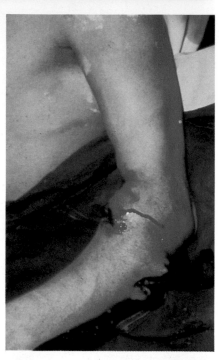 **A penetrating and destructive injury caused by an explosive type of accident at work.**

132 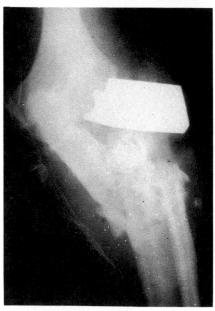 **In spite of the loss of parts of the radius, extensor muscles and the radial nerve,** the man regained a remarkably good elbow after extensive toilet and internal fixation.

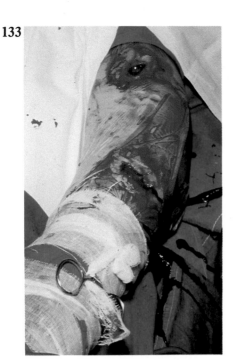

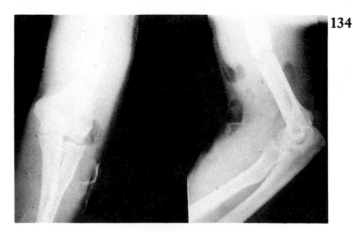

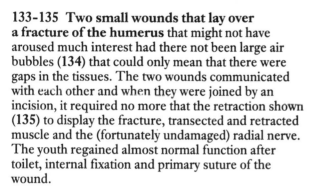

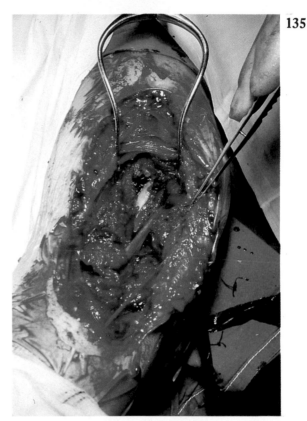

133-135 Two small wounds that lay over a fracture of the humerus that might not have aroused much interest had there not been large air bubbles (134) that could only mean that there were gaps in the tissues. The two wounds communicated with each other and when they were joined by an incision, it required no more that the retraction shown (135) to display the fracture, transected and retracted muscle and the (fortunately undamaged) radial nerve. The youth regained almost normal function after toilet, internal fixation and primary suture of the wound.

136 A fairly short-range shotgun wound of the forearm. The shot had begun to scatter and some of the pellets came to lie under the skin on the other side of the limb. The entire flexor digitorum superficialis had to be removed and a damaged segment of the radial artery was bypassed. Later, a cable graft was let into the median nerve and the patient regained very useful function.

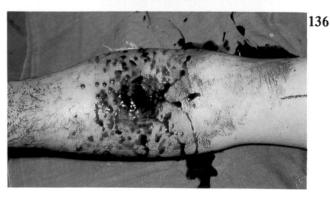

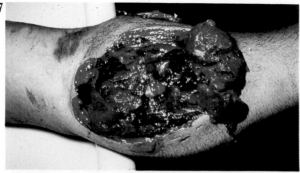

137 The exit wound caused by a powerful shotgun fired at short range.

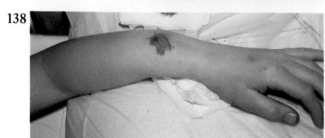

138 An open fracture showing penetration from within by a spike of bone, which is unusual in a child.

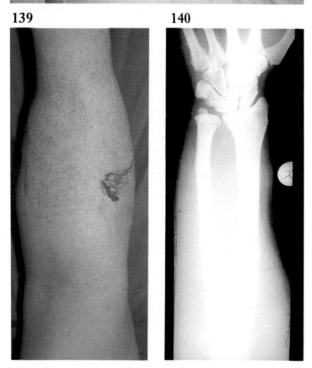

139 Penetration of the forearm caused by a nailgun; the nail went through the limb.

140 The splintered radius remained stable.

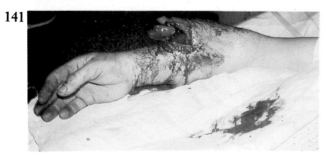

141 A severe open fracture that tore through all the extensor muscles. In spite of the dusky appearance of the hand (which was caused largely by dirt), the main nerve and blood supplies were intact. Also, in spite of infection and other complications after toilet, primary internal fixation and closure, the man retained his morale and regained use of his hand.

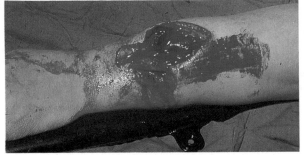

142 **With less forcible injury, the bones may erupt between muscles and tendons;** their ends can be seen resting on the distal skin edge. In this case, the only muscle that needed to be repaired was extensor pollicis longus; the others had been parted by the bones.

Comment If both bones come out of a single wound there is no objection to extending it, if necessary, so as to allow both bones to be fixed through the one incision.

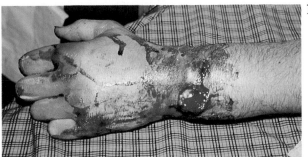

143 **Fracture-dislocation of the inferior radioulnar joint,** with the lower end of the ulna sticking out. Note the marked swelling of the hand, which also affected the palm. Both surfaces of the hand were decompressed by generous incisions and the radioulnar joint was temporarily secured with a Kirschner's wire. There was full recovery.

Comment Massive swelling of the hand can lead to severe and lasting stiffness; evacuation of the haematoma may prevent this and should be carried out as soon as possible.

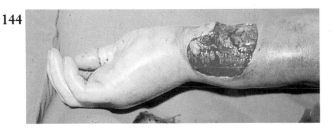

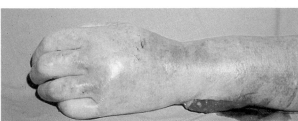

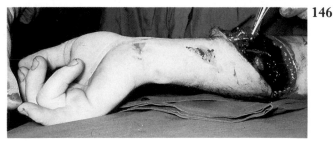

144 and 145 **This injury was inflicted when the wrist was caught between rollers;** note the badly swollen hand. In spite of evacuation of the blood and the use of suction drainage, the patient—an elderly woman—never recovered full extension of her fingers; there may have been damage to the muscles.

146 **This forearm was cut to the bone in front and bled freely from the severed arteries.** Identification of the distal ends of muscles and tendons is much easier if the fingers are exposed when the wound is explored. The tendon being tested was flexing the tip of the little finger.

Comment The less the cut surfaces are disturbed by dissection, the less the normal relationships of the structures are altered and the less are the difficulties of identification. A clear knowledge of the cross-sectional anatomy is necessary; diagrams or textbooks should be referred to in case of doubt. Not all structures that retract do so up well-defined tunnels, but their passage is usually marked by traces of blood. Some can be 'milked' down, others can be found by the careful use of fine retractors, accurate knowledge and a good light. Formal dissection is not usually necessary and careless dissection can be disastrous.

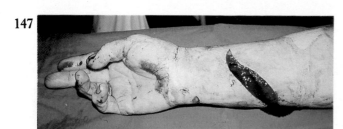

147 Although the wound appeared to affect the ulnar side of the forearm, it had penetrated far enough to the radial side to cut both flexor tendons of the fore and middle fingers and the superficial flexor of the ring finger, as was shown by the fact that the tip of the ring finger was still flexed.

Comment The natural resting posture of the hand is maintained under general anaesthesia and after paralysing drugs. Any alteration of the posture is the result of damage to muscles, tendons or nerves.

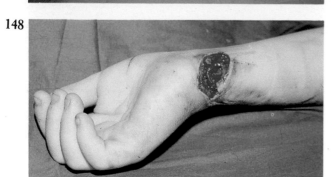

148 This wound damaged the ulnar nerve but none of the tendons. At this level posture will not be affected but the intrinsic muscles will be paralysed and part of the hand will be numb and not sweating.

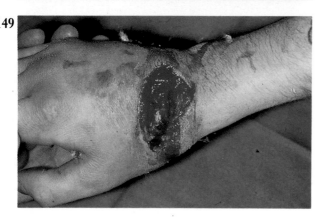

149 A grinding injury that divided the tendons of extensores pollicis longus et carpi radialis longus and also deposited rusty grit in the carpus. Nevertheless, the wound healed uneventfully after irrigation, toilet and a split skin graft. The tendon of extensor indicis was later transferred through a tunnel created under the split skin graft with the aid of a silicone rod.

Swelling and deformity

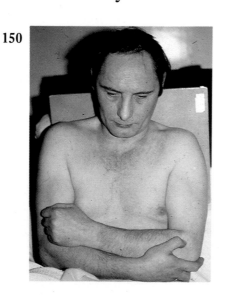

The clavicle

150 A characteristic posture in which the sound limb supports the injured one. There was no visible deformity but there was slight swelling over a fracture at the medial end of the left clavicle.

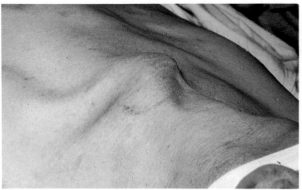

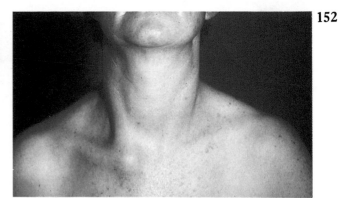

151 Fracture at the inner end of the left clavicle, seen from above the left shoulder. The sharpness of the prominence distinguished this from **anterior dislocation of the sternoclavicular joint—152.**

153 Posterior dislocation of the medial end of the clavicle is rare. It follows a heavy blow or a fall that drives the shoulder inwards and forwards. The inner end of the clavicle sometimes presses on the trachea or a large blood vessel in the neck. The loss of the normal prominence of the left clavicle could be seen both from the front and also on looking down at the shoulders. Unlike anterior dislocation, this is stable when corrected.

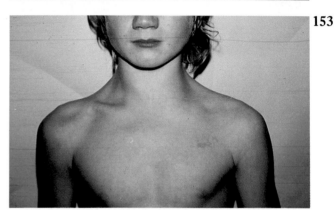

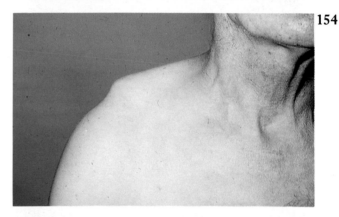

154 The dislocation of the acromioclavicular joint was obvious. Contrary to what is often stated, the clavicle is not pulled up; the forequarter drops under its own weight and the scapula also slides forwards round the ribs. The deformity can be corrected if the victim braces back the shoulder.

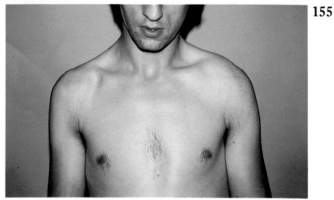

155 In this case, displacement of the acromio-clavicular joint was masked by swelling, but there were marks of impact just behind the shoulder.

The shoulder joint

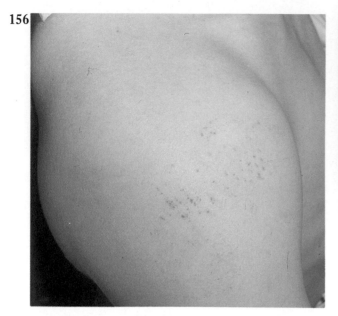

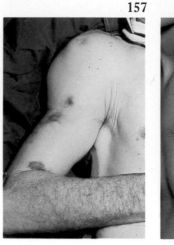

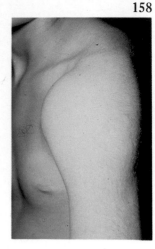

156 The right shoulder is viewed from the right side. The general swelling shown was caused by an effusion into the shoulder joint following a fracture of the glenoid cavity; the marks of impact can be seen.

157 An example of the more extensive swelling caused by an effusion of blood, but in this case note that the general line of the arm pointed towards the neck; that was because there was a dislocation as well as a fracture.

158 Greenstick fracture. The slight general swelling of this shoulder was accompanied by a forward prominence that was caused by a greenstick fracture of the neck of the humerus.

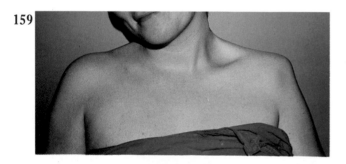

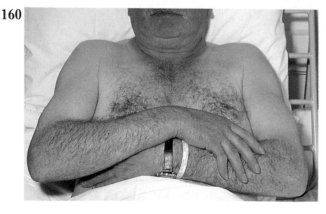

159 Anterior dislocation of the shoulder. The flattening of the outer side of the left shoulder with resulting angularity that is typical of anterior dislocation; bruising and swelling may appear later. The inward inclination of the upper end of the humerus was not very obvious in this case.

160 Anterior dislocation of the shoulder. The well-muscled and the fat have less obvious deformity and the shape of this bulky man's shoulder looks normal. Nevertheless, the line of the arm can be seen to be inclined slightly inwards at its upper end. The dislocated head of the humerus was responsible for the congestion of the veins in the right arm.

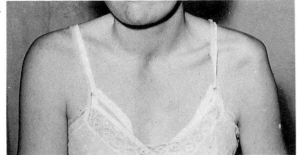

161 The left shoulder showed downward subluxation resulting from long-standing muscular weakness—note the hollow beneath the clavicle. Voluntary correction was possible.

162 This patient's left shoulder had been dislocated for 4 months. The abduction shown was mostly the result of rotation of the scapula.

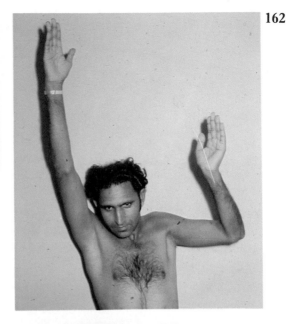

162

163 Posterior dislocation of the shoulder is rare and is easily overlooked. As well as pain and loss of movement, the humerus is held in medial rotation but this is likely to be taken to be the natural resting posture of the limb. The fact that the xray appearances are not usually obviously abnormal adds to the difficulty in diagnosis.

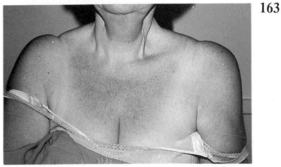

163

164 The discerning eye and fingers will recognise the loss of the normal fullness of the front of the shoulder and a prominence at the back. The palpable loss of the normal anterior prominence has been mistaken for a soft, cystic swelling.

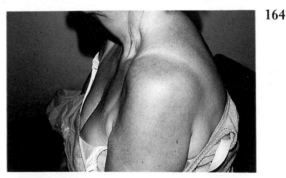

164

165 The alteration in shape is often most easily recognised by looking at the shoulders from above. In this case, the right shoulder was the dislocated one. The condition had gone unrecognised for a month. It has been known for a patient with a posterior dislocation to be sent to the physiotherapy department with a diagnosis of frozen shoulder and for a physiotherapist to suspect the true condition. The appearance of an anteroposterior xray was not very helpful in this case.

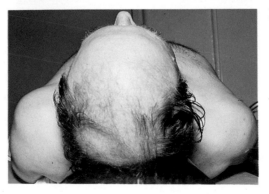

165

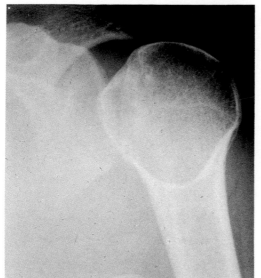

166 Posterior dislocation of the shoulder. In this shoulder the complete ring of cortical bone in the head of the humerus was caused by the fixed medial rotation of the dislocated humerus. This is a useful warning and it will also be noted that the notch between the tuberosities of the humerus can be seen. An axillary view shows this dislocation clearly but it may not be possible because of pain and stiffness; a lateral view taken through the chest is not easy to interpret.

Comment Like anterior dislocation, posterior dislocation can be recurrent; in those with lax joints this may be precipitated by a very mild injury and recur very easily.

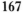

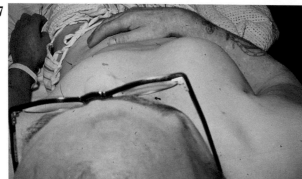

Torn muscles
167 This man was trapped when a brick furnace collapsed on him while he was helping to repair it. His alarming appearance on reaching hospital (caused by blood and brick dust, *see* **440**) responded well to soap and water. On looking down from above, the prominence of the right breast and hollowness of the anterior axillary region were striking. The pectoralis major had been crushed through and had retracted medially.

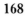

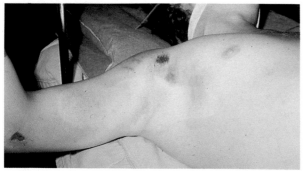

168 A similar injury had occurred in this case but the deformity was hidden by swelling. However, the gap in the muscle could be felt easily.

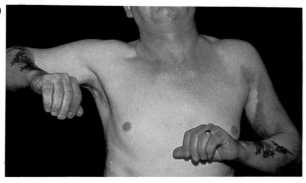

169 Extensive rupture of the rotator cuff of the left shoulder had removed the means of initiating abduction. The widespread bruising with little swelling and no deformity of the shoulder made fracture or dislocation unlikely.

The arm and elbow
Rupture of the tendon of the long head of the biceps is well known.

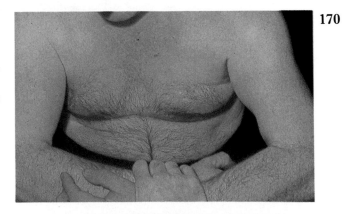

170 Avulsion of the lower end is rare. Bending the elbow and supinating the forearm against resistance caused the belly of the muscle to form a ball just above the middle of the arm.

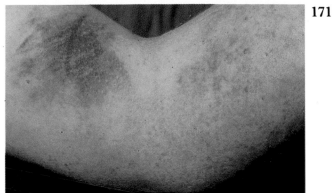

171 There was also bruising near the elbow. Because the whole muscle is rendered ineffective, this is a much more disabling condition than rupture of the long head and the tendon should be stitched back.

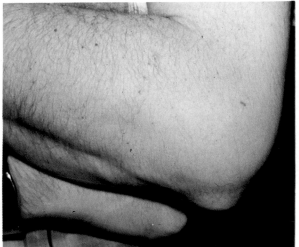

172 The whole elbow was swollen and very painful and it was acutely tender over the lateral epicondyle of the humerus, where there was ectopic calcification. This is a rare condition analogous with acute calcification in the rotator cuff of the shoulder.

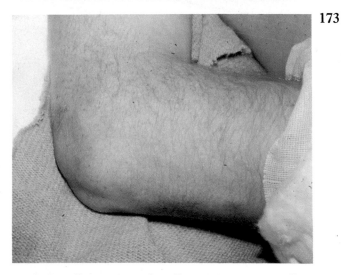

173 An effusion into the elbow joint can usually be identified by the swelling that it produces over the radiohumeral joint and is well shown here. An effusion is often evidence of a fracture but in this case it was the result of a blow that did not cause a fracture.

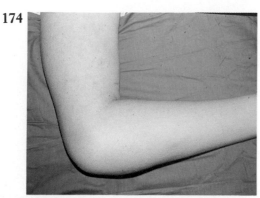

174 The whole elbow looked slightly swollen but was not otherwise misshapen. There was a mild fracture of the olecranon process of the ulna, caused by a fall on to the point of the elbow.

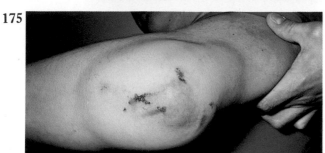

175 This fracture of the olecranon process was also caused by a fall and was accompanied by more evident damage. (Looking towards the point of the bent elbow; the shoulder is to the right.)

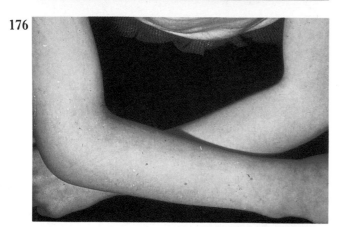

176 Mild general swelling of the elbow that was caused by a supracondylar fracture of the right humerus. Unlike the two previous cases, this followed a fall on to the outstretched hand. The difference between the histories is important.

Comment A slight prominence at the back of the elbow after a fall on to the hand might be the result of either dislocation or a mild supracondylar fracture.

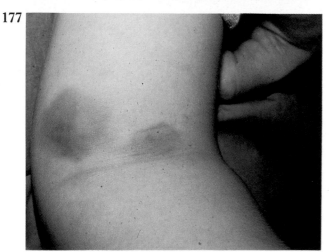

177 When there is a fracture with much displacement, there is often bruising on the inner side of the front of the elbow, where the bone is sometimes prominent enough to blanch the skin or even pierce it. The left elbow is shown.

178 Posterior dislocation of the elbow joint with marked deformity.

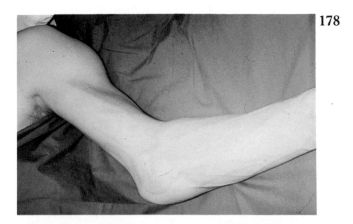

179 An unusual variety of fracture-subluxation in which the displacement of the forearm was medial. The mark caused by the heavy blow that was responsible is clearly visible. (Shoulder on left; hand on right.)

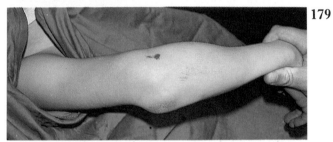

180 Lateral displacement of the forearm with dislocation of the elbow occurs more often than medial. Until they have been obliterated by progressive swelling, the prominence of the head of the radius and the hollow above it are characteristic of this type of dislocation.

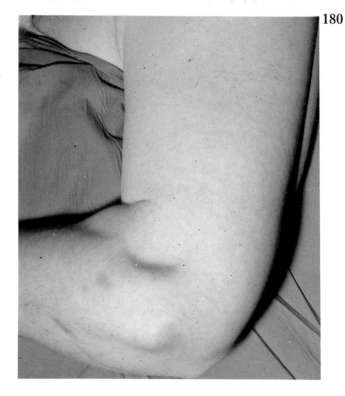

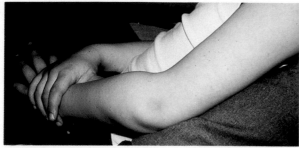

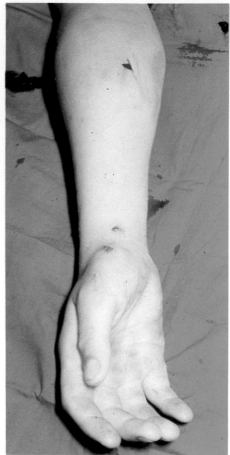

181 The discerning eye may recognise that this was a mild example of the anterior type of Monteggia's fracture-subluxation. There is lateral prominence of the displaced head of the radius with a hollow behind it and swelling over the ulna. However, the main purpose of the photograph is to show that what may seem to be thoughtless neglect to apply a sling and a plaster of Paris slab was in fact considerate agreement to the boy's request to be allowed to go on holding the limb himself, which he continued to do even after falling asleep on his father's lap. The patient may know better than the doctor or the nurse in other cases as well.

182 A Monteggia injury with which not much deformity was evident but there was obvious anterior swelling. The small wound on the front of the forearm was made by the proximal fragment of the ulna, which was sharply cocked up. In children, many of these injuries can be treated successfully by fixing the forearm in full supination in a plaster cast extending from the deltoid muscle to the knuckles. However, when the proximal end of the ulna is cocked up as much as it was in this case, it may be trapped in the muscles and require an operation to release it and then to fix it. Internal fixation is almost always necessary in adults. (The marks at the base of the thumb were caused by falling on to the hand.) Monteggia's injury is a variation of dislocation of the elbow in which the ulna remains in place against the humerus but, by breaking, it allows the radius to slip either forwards or backwards out of joint. The anterior injury can also occur as a result of violent and excessive pronation.

183 This Monteggia injury followed a blow, the mark of which is clearly shown, together with the characteristic deformity. The hand was resting on the board and pad. When the hand was lifted against gravity, the slight ridge made by extensor carpi radialis longus could be seen more clearly than in the photograph. No other extensor muscle was acting because they are all supplied by the posterior interosseous nerve, which is sometimes damaged by the displaced head of the radius. Extensor carpi radialis longus is supplied by the main trunk of the radial nerve, which is not at risk. The fact that there is no wrist drop can cause the fact that the posterior interosseous nerve has been damaged to go unrecognised, as at first it did in this case. Unless this complication of Monteggia's injury is known, it will not be looked for with due care.

There was also a fracture of the shaft of the

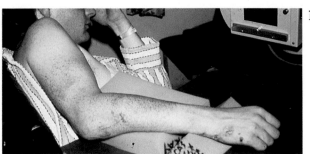

183

humerus and the mark of impact can be seen. Both fractures were plated within a few hours and the limb recovered fully in all respects. If it is not recognised and operation is not carried out until the next convenient list, the paralysis that results may be permanent.

184 This bony injury resembled the one in 183, except that it was accompanied by extensive, deep burns. The fractures were fixed at once. There is no objection to operating through freshly burned skin, which should be prepared as though it were normal and if necessary replaced by grafts later. If the burns become infected, the deeper tissues have usually become sealed off from the skin and remain free from infection.

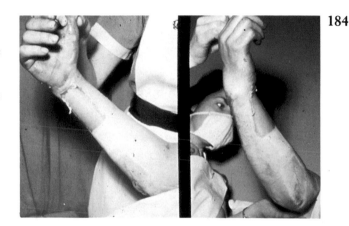

184

The wrist

185 This deformity looks like a mild Colles's fracture but a serious and complicated fracture-dislocation of the wrist caused swelling rather than deformity.

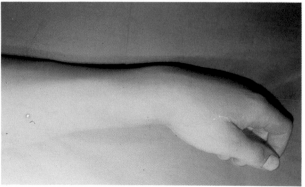

185

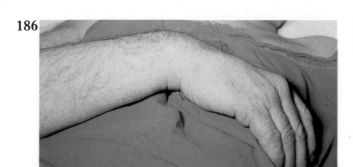

186 As seen from the side, this severe example of Smith's fracture was not remarkable.

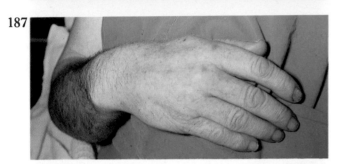

187 When seen from the back the prominence of the ulna caused by the displacement of the radius was well shown.

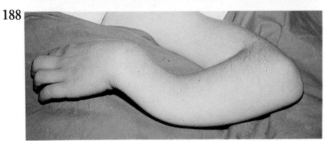

188 A greenstick fracture with marked deformity.

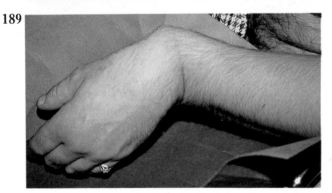

189 A severe and unusual fracture of the radius with disruption of the inferior radioulnar joint.

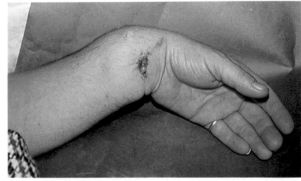

190 The jagged edge of the radius nearly broke through the skin. The median nerve had escaped damage in this case.

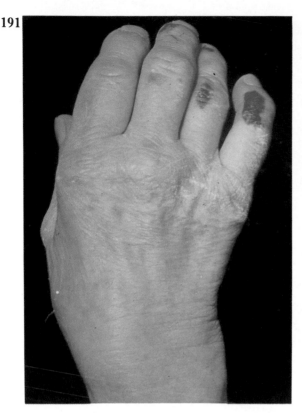

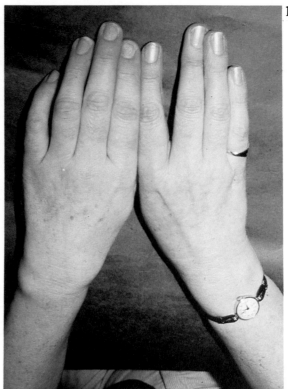

191 Although the hand looked a little gnarled, the swelling over the lower end of the radius was not the result of arthritis but followed a fall. The swelling was at first confined to the line of the tendon of extensor pollicis longus. The cause was an effusion of blood into the sheath of that tendon from an underlying crack in the bone. Within a few hours the swelling had spread more widely and was no longer of any particular diagnostic value.

192 In this case the swelling was limited proximally by the extensor retinaculum. Unless the wrist is examined carefully the swelling may be thought to be in the anatomical snuffbox, whereas at first it forms one of its boundaries. Later it spreads out.

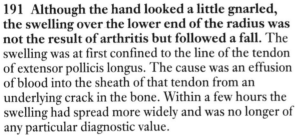

193 When swelling in the anatomical snuffbox follows a fall or a forcible wrench, it is usually regarded as evidence of a fracture of the scaphoid bone; this is often the case but it is not the fracture but the effusion of blood from it that causes the swelling. Swelling in the anatomical snuffbox is evidence of an effusion into the radiocarpal joint and is not necessarily the result of a fracture, or even injury. One consequence of the ingrained belief that swelling in the snuffbox equals fracture of the scaphoid bone is repeated radiography and prolonged use of plaster of Paris in the belief that because the wrist remains weak, stiff and painful, a fracture must be present even though it cannot be identified with xrays. Two causes of such confusion are Bennett's fracture-subluxation and tearing of the scapholunate ligament. Normally, when there is a clear space between the scaphoid and lunate bones it is not more

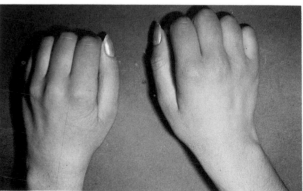

than 2-3 mm wide; any more than this is evidence of rupture. This can occur as a result of a fall on to the hand, spontaneously as a result of attrition or as part of a disruptive lesion of the carpus.

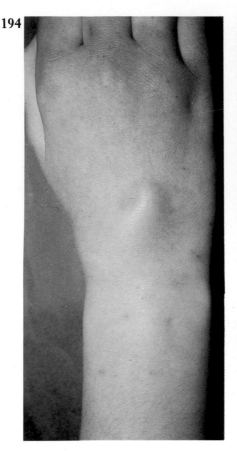

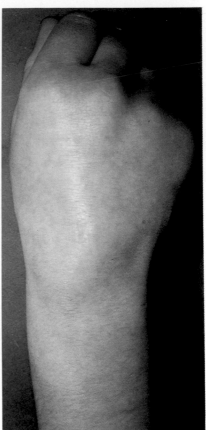

194 This bluish, tender and tensely cystic dorsal swelling followed a fall on to the hand. It was caused by an effusion of blood along the tendons of extensores carpi radiales longus et brevis from an underlying crack in the radius.

195 Such a swelling soon spreads out. The explanation of these appearances is that because the fracture is small in extent and mild in degree, there is little damage to the adjoining soft tissues. The effusion first takes the line of least resistance, which in these cases was into the overlying tendons' sheaths or paratenon.

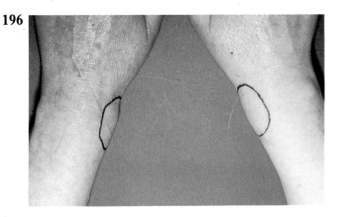

196 De Quervain's so-called tenovaginitis stenosans is not easy to diagnose in its early stages because there is not much swelling or tenderness and symptoms are little more than aching or twinges when using the hand. Once it has been fixed clearly in the mind's eye, the swelling (on the left wrist), though not large, is characteristic in shape and position; tenderness is accurately confined to the swelling and flexion of the thumb when the wrist is bent to the ulnar side is painful. In fairness to the patient, who is usually female, this test should be applied gently.

5 The hand

Wounds

Wounds of the hand have been divided usefully into tidy and untidy groups. Tidy wounds are for the most part pricks, punctures and incised wounds, including clean amputations. Untidy wounds are lacerated, contused and often complex.

Pricks and punctures

No structure in the hand is more than about half an inch from the surface. When the fist is clenched, the soft tissues on the dorsal aspects of the joints are no more than 2 or 3 mm thick. Any dorsal wound over the joint should be examined with the possibility of penetration in mind. The phrase, 'I knocked my hand at work', may indicate a much more forceful injury than the often nonchalant tone in which it is described may lead one to suspect. Useful additional warnings are the oozing of synovial liquid from the wound or the presence of air in the joint. Unless penetration can certainly be ruled out, be prepared to explore any joint about which ones suspicions have been aroused. Exploration must be carried out with the joint in all positions of flexion and extension, before declaring it not to have been opened.

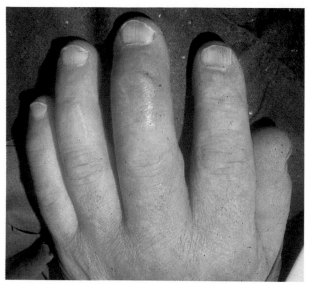

197

197 This man knocked his finger at work but he did nothing about it for a fortnight although it was still rather sore. Dusky swelling and the fine groove of a scar near the base of the nail suggested that there was grumbling infection in the terminal joint and xrays confirmed this.

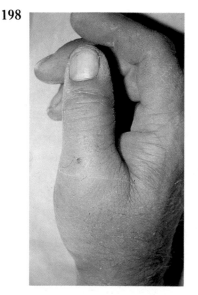

198

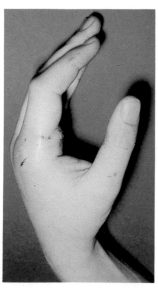

199

198 This man sought advice after pricking his thumb while gardening. Exploration discovered a tiny thorn that had just entered the joint. In spite of the slightly turbid exudate, the wound healed promptly after irrigation and the joint recovered fully.

199 Within a few hours of being bitten by his cat, the pain in his finger brought this man to hospital. Figure **200** shows the appearance inside the joint.

63

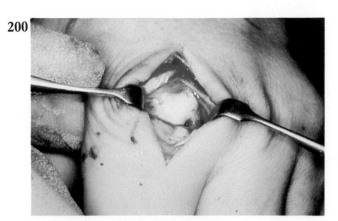

200 When it was explored from the dorsum, the joint contained turbid blood. The mark of a tooth could be seen on the head of the metacarpal, which is shown just to the right of the left hand retractor. The hand is partly clenched and is viewed from beyond the knuckles; the wrist is above and the fingers are below. In spite of bony defects that were radiologically obvious 5 months later, the joint had recovered fully. It had closed spontaneously after being irrigated by means of a fine drip-feed for 2 days.

Comment (i) Unless there is obviously established infection, it is probably sufficient to wash out the joint with penicillin (to which Past. multocida, the usual germ implanted by cats' teeth, is sensitive), close it and give one or two more doses by mouth or by injection.
(ii) Cats' teeth can also implant germs under the extensor tendons or expansions; all such bites on the hand require careful and speedy treatment.

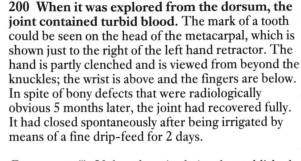

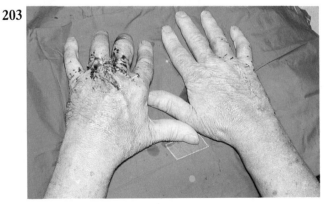

201 The right thumb had been bitten by a dog 3 weeks before; the swollen segment contained a fracture that had gone unsuspected for that length of time.

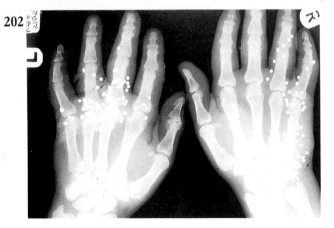

202 So many pellets might be expected to inflict severe damage, but the only ones that were removed were those found in a wound leading into the left third metacarpophalangeal joint and those that later became troublesome lumps under the skin.

203 The appearance of the hands 13 days after being injured. The right hand recovered fully; the left middle and ring fingers were rather stiff.

Comment The pellets came from a bird-scarer and travelled much more slowly than those from a shotgun; they did correspondingly less damage.

Injury by injection

Many substances are now forced through fine nozzles by pressures varying from hundreds to thousands of pounds per square inch. With the exception of water, which is absorbed, and some plastic materials that solidify, all the injected material cannot be removed and what remains within the tissues acts as a potent irritant. To the damage done by inflammation may be added the ischaemic effects of tight distension of the part, when the injecting pressure is high.

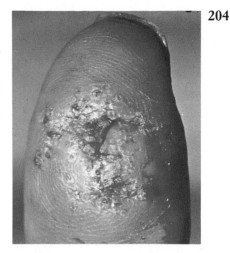

204 About a teaspoonful of grease had been injected into the fingertip, which became almost useless because of scarring in spite of prompt evacuation of all recognisable grease.

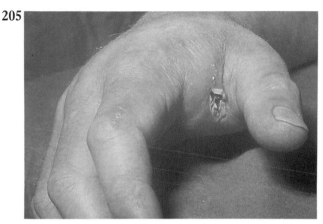

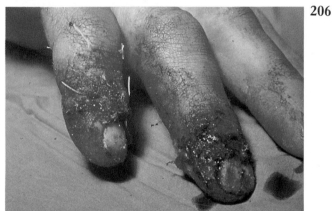

205 A fairly large amount of paraffin was injected into this hand. A few days after generous incision the wound was badly inflamed; the forefinger died and had to be amputated a few days later.

Fingertips

206 and 207 The severity of these injuries was apparently underestimated, until xrays (**207**) were made some days after stitches were inserted.

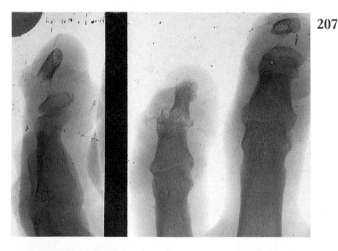

Comment The painful, injured finger must be xrayed, because both the external appearances and the account of the accident can be seriously misleading.

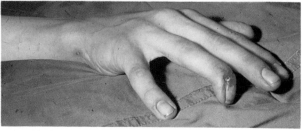

208 When the nail has been uprooted it may mean that there has been a fracture at the base of the terminal phalanx. In this case, the sharp bend was not at the joint but at a fracture through the base of the terminal phalanx.

65

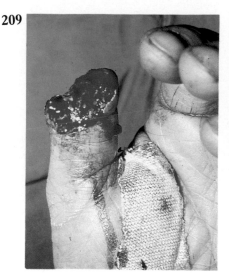

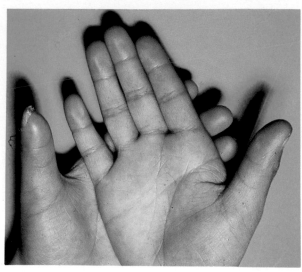

209 Amputations of the fingertip that spare all or most of the pulp can be dealt with very well by free or flap grafts. If there is persistent bleeding, grafting can be deferred for a day or two without detriment to the result.

210 In children, loss of the fingertip usually heals with a small scar, whether grafted or merely dressed and left to heal, as the left thumb was. It provided a satisfactory working surface with the ability both to hold and to open a safety pin with the eyes closed.

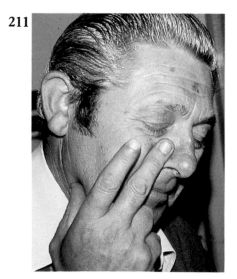

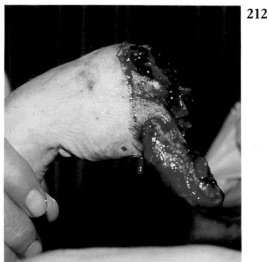

211 In an adult, the neatest looking fingertip will go unused if it lacks tactile gnosis. This man underwent an apparently successful Kutler's repair of the forefinger, but he used the middle finger to scratch his face.

212 A case in which the partly severed thumb and 2 fingers were suitable for reattachment. In spite of such a distressing injury, the patient was able to discuss the recommended treatment before deciding to accept it.

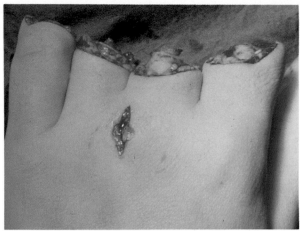

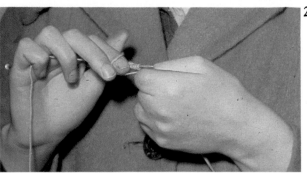

214 The unselfconscious and successful way in which this woman used her hand did much to distract attention from her loss of fingers. However, not all patients adjust as well as she did.

Comment The fact that existing skin can be drawn together over bone does not necessarily mean that this should be done; if the skin is tight, this is like having a dressing that is too tight and the stump is unlikely to be usable once it has healed.

213 Bone was protruding from these finger stumps because the skin had retracted; the skin was trimmed to shape and the resulting flaps were sewn up easily.

Cut tendons

215 Tendons can be cut through smaller wounds than the one shown. Even under general anaesthesia and with full relaxation, the natural resting posture of the part is altered if a tendon has been cut (*see* **147**). Active flexion confirmed that flexor digitorum profundus had been cut but the fact that flexor superficialis was acting did not mean that it had escaped damage. In such a case, exploration must be carried out and the tendon watched throughout its full excursion. If it has been more than half divided, it should be repaired or at least protected from risk of later rupture by splinting so as to prevent tension on it for a few weeks.

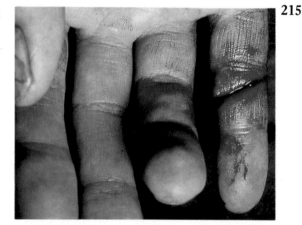

215

216 A penetrating wound of the hypothenar eminence had cut both flexor tendons of the little finger, but there was slight flexor tone at the meta-carpophalangeal joint. The hand was palm upwards when photographed.

Comment Even in an unco-operative child the nerves and tendons can be tested by the judicious (and concealed) use of a pin, which shows whether or not the finger is sensible and whether or not the action of withdrawal is carried out at all the usual joints.

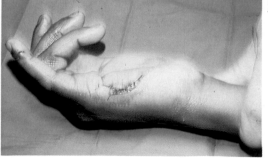

216

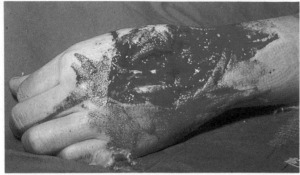

217

217 This untidy wound had extended into the bones of the carpus as well as dividing the extensor tendons. As a result, under the influence of gravity, the hand was unduly flexed at the wrist.

Grinding and crushing

These injuries are usually inflicted by rollers or heavy weights, which are sometimes combined. Light contact with rapidly rotating objects results in friction burns, which usually heal well. Heavier pressure removes or crushes the skin but the resulting appearance is not always a reliable guide to the outcome. Heavy pressure splits and tears the skin from the tissues beneath and can be severely destructive; nevertheless, remarkable healing and recovery can occur.

218

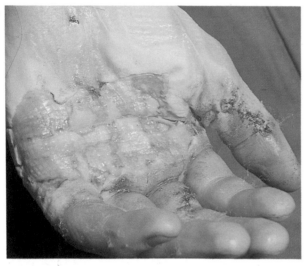

218 Superficial friction burns of the palm about 10 days after injury. The back of the hand was similarly affected. The badly swollen hand was decompressed promptly. Suction drainage and elevation in a firm dressing all helped to prevent recurrent swelling. The hand healed spontaneously and full function was restored.

Comment A friction burn that destroys skin and tendons and exposes bone may require immediate application of a flap graft.

21

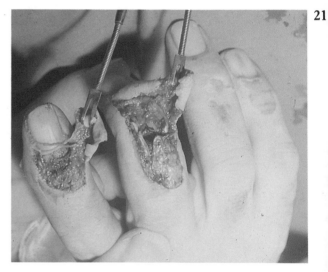

219 Local destruction by grinding. The extensor tendon of the forefinger had been ground away and the joint was open. In the middle finger much of the bone had been ground away; reconstruction was technically possible but offered little functional advantage.

220 The man agreed to amputation but there was enough skin to close both wounds, using the middle finger to provide a primary tube for the forefinger. The forefingertip was stiff but very useful.

Comment Viable tissue from one injured part may be put to better use in the restoration of another part than in local reconstruction or conservation.

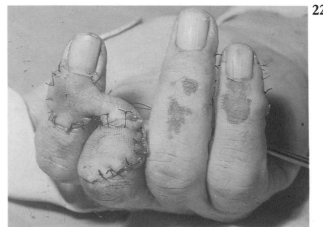

220

221 Severe friction burn in a child who had been knocked from his bicycle. The carpus had been opened and part of the hypothenar eminence had been ground away. Split skin was applied to the hand immediately after surgical toilet and to the forearm later, when it was evidently necessary.

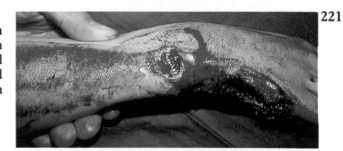

221

222

222 As seemed likely on the first examination, three fingers (fore, middle and ring) could not be saved and delayed primary amputation was carried out. In this case the friction was accompanied by fairly heavy crushing.

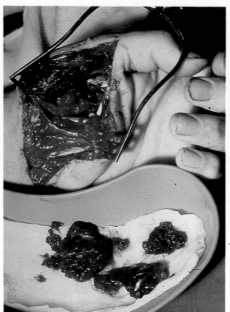

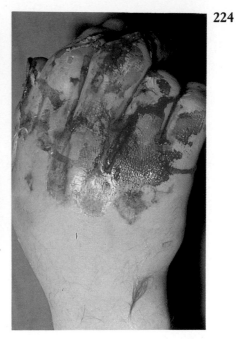

223 A small dorsal wound was accompanied by a severe wound of the base of the palm, here seen laid open, with pulped muscle that had been cut away, mostly from the thenar group of muscles. Xrays showed air in the wound as well as the fracture.

224 The appearance of the skin near the middle of the metacarpus is characteristic of what might be described as a crush-bruise.

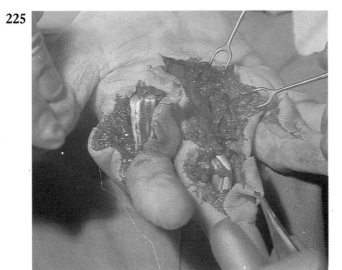

225 The palm was severely torn but no bone was broken, two fingers were lost but the crushed skin recovered unexpectedly well.

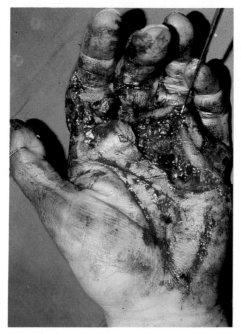

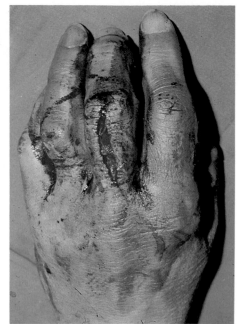

226 and 227 In spite of the initial appearance, this hand recovered fully after no more than surgical toilet and closure (227); there was no fracture. The discoloration was caused by dirt, not ischaemia from crushing.

Comment Because it can at first be very difficult to predict the outcome of an injury, there is a place for cautious optimism when important parts may still be viable.

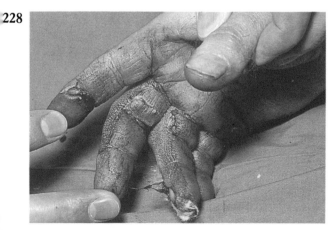

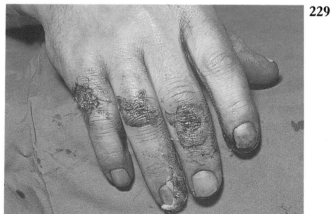

228 and 229 These fingers were caught in machinery. Although they did not look serious, the fact that there were wounds on both palmar and dorsal surfaces suggested that the intervening structures had also been damaged. Xrays confirmed this assumption and showed nearly right-angled deformity near the distal ends of the middle phalanges of the ring and little fingers.

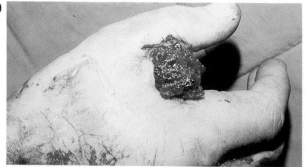

230 An unusual result of crushing; interosseous muscle had been torn from the bone and forced out of a split in the web. The muscle neither twitched nor bled and was removed. In spite of the defect, a good range of abduction of the first metacarpal was possible.

Comment If dead muscle is not removed, and especially if it becomes infected, the subsequent scarring may severely restrict movements. Without the clogging effect of such a scar, remarkable recovery of function can occur.

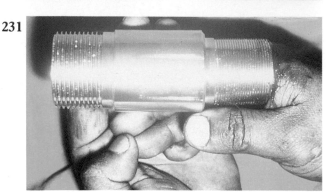

231 An unusual injury of the forefinger. The heavy brass casting (which the employers were pleased to have back) could be unscrewed from the finger only with analgaesia. Although the skin of the finger had acquired a male thread and was not expected to survive, it recovered well. Eight-and-a-half months later there was full extension and nearly full flexion, with normal sensibility.

Avulsion and flaying

Avulsion can occur as a result of a straight pull or as part of a crushing and stripping injury. In some cases, survival of the stripped skin is unexpectedly good, so an initially conservative operation should be considered.

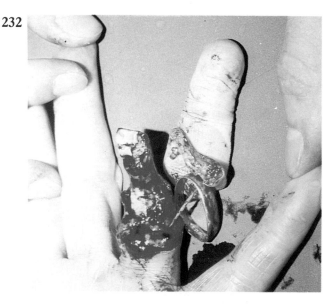

232 A typical ring avulsion injury. Reconstruction is possible but amputation should be advised.

233 Tendons may be avulsed from bone or through their motors. This man's hand was trapped by a metal band in a machine used for securing large packages and was subjected to a strong pulling action that disorganised the carpometacarpal joints. The wound went most of the way round the wrist. The part shown here was on the radial side of the wrist and the base of the thumb, which is on the right. The significance of the sagging tendons on the radial side of the wrist was not at first understood, in spite of the fact that it could be seen that a tendon had been torn out. The explanation came to mind while the author was shaving and was confirmed by exploration.

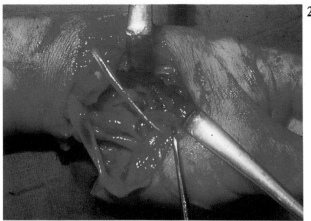

234 Torn extensor, abductor and flexor pollicis longus. When the forearm was explored, it was found that the bellies of extensor, abductor and flexor pollicis longus had been torn through. (The hand is above the right edge of the photograph.) While they were still within their intact fascial sheaths the muscles appeared to have been no more than bruised, but once the blood had been evacuated the gaps in the muscle bellies were revealed.

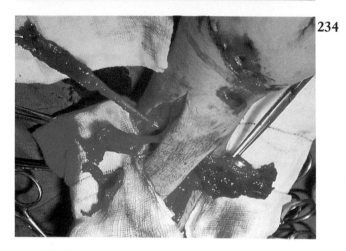

235 The dusky appearance of this retrograde avulsion flap bodes ill but after toilet and suture the wound healed without need of a graft.

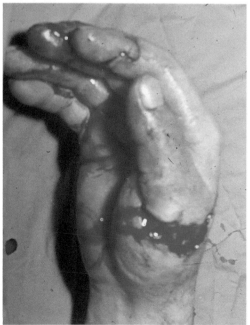

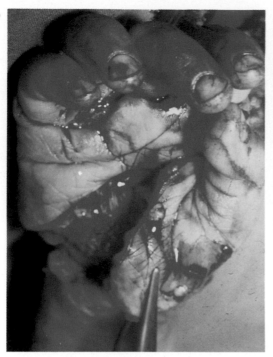

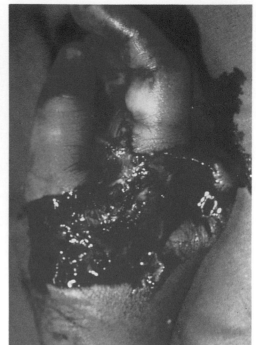

236 and **237 A little boy's hand was run over in the road.** Although the large and untidy flaps were pink throughout and bled briskly from their edges, little of the skin survived (**237**). Delayed primary amputation and skin grafting yielded a very useful extremity that was later improved by releasing a contracture of the thumb.

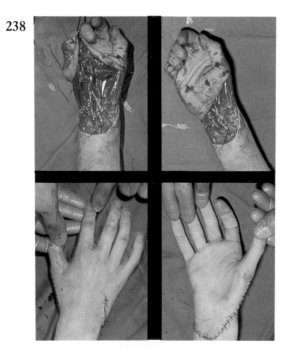

238 The palmar skin and fat were torn loose almost to the metacarpophalangeal joints, leaving the deeper structures largely intact. However ill-judged it might be thought to be to have sewn this skin back, nearly all of it survived.

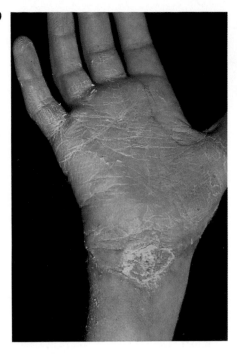

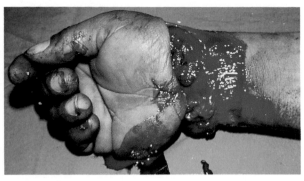

240 Extensively flayed palm. The first appearance of the hand of a 28-year-old man. The palm had been flayed almost as extensively as in the last case and it healed as well after simple toilet and suture.

Comment (i) Suction drainage, a snug dressing and elevation are necessary after sewing back skin flaps. (ii) The practice of replacing large flaps of skin has long been condemned but when the skin is as specialised as that of the palm, its survival is to the great advantage of the patient and is by no means impossible. If the primary surgical toilet is carried out carefully but the flap dies, infection is unusual. It is often possible to apply grafts immediately after removing the dead tissue.

239 The small graft that was required on the front of the wrist can be seen. Full function was recovered.

241 and 242 Same hand as shown in 236 and 237, 3 weeks before. Immediately after removing the dead tissue it was possible to apply dermatome grafts to the raw surfaces, where they took well.

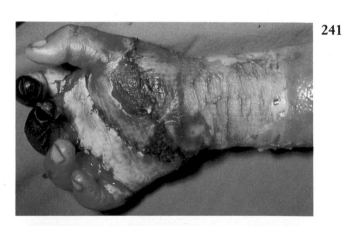

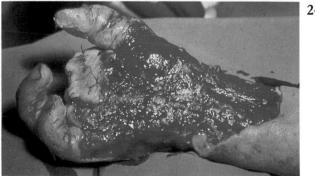

Complex wounds

Such wounds can tax the ingenuity and skill of the most experienced surgeon and may require numerous stages of reconstruction over the course of months or even years. On the other hand, essentially simple surgical measures can sometimes enable one operation to be enough. The judgement, foresight and technical skill required are now so widely available that there is no need to hesitate to transfer patients after consultation with suitable centres.

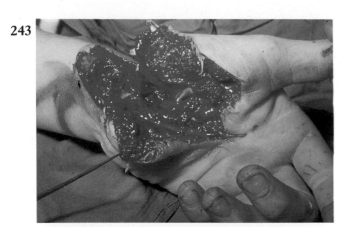

243 The wound itself was more informative than the xray appearance after a saw cut deeply and obliquely into the carpus, severing flexor tendons, the median nerve and the deep branch of the ulnar nerve. Complete primary repair yielded a usable hand.

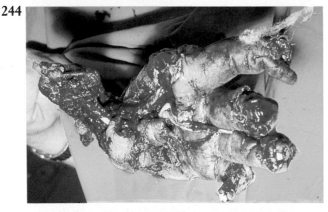

244 This is the result of playing with gunpowder. What remained viable could be determined only by careful examination under anaesthesia, first with and then without a tourniquet.

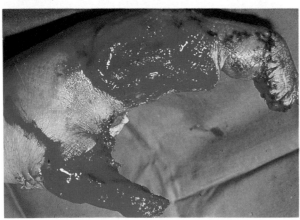

245 What remained of the hand was ready for split skin grafting 4 days later.

246 Internal fixation maintained a shape that enabled a determined and courageous young man to use the stumps as forceps. Some months after returning to work he required one further operation to release a contracture and add sensibility to the remnant of his thumb by means of an island flap.

Comment (i) When several stages of reconstruction are required, it is to the patient's advantage if the hand can be put to some use between each stage.
(ii) Injuries of this sort understandably arouse a good deal of interest and require the attention of someone more experienced than the emergency room officer who first sees it. Nevertheless, every effort should be made to minimise the number of times that the dressing is removed to allow inspection.

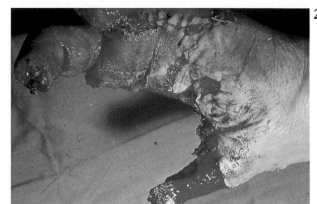

246

Infection

Most infections of the hand follow wounds which may be small enough to be disregarded at first. Serious infections are now rare and most likely to follow large or neglected wounds.

247 A typical infection of the pulp, for which prompt evacuation of all pus and obliteration of a healthy cavity allows healing in 7-10 days, without need for antibiotics.

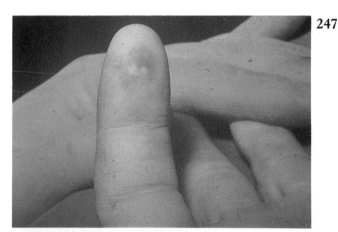

247

248 The forefinger was the infected one.
Although the 'point' of the abscess (in the proximal interphalangeal crease) was small, the whole finger was swollen and slightly straighter than the others. This suggested that the flexor tendons' sheath had been affected. In most forefingers this sheath extends only as far as the palm but in a few it reaches as far as the wrist, with correspondingly situated swelling and tenderness. Movement of the finger was possible but much restricted by pain.

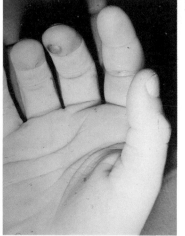

248

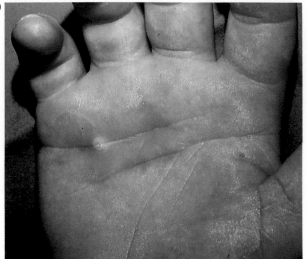

249 Pus pointing in the palm may signify a superficial abscess, as was suggested in this case by the fairly small area of redness, tenderness and swelling, but it can occur with a subfascial (collar stud) abscess that has reached the surface. Therefore, a deep source of infection must be remembered and sought when the abscess is incised.

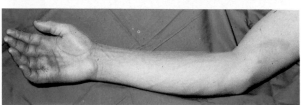

250 A large palmar abscess with lymphangitis; an antibiotic should be given before drainage and for a day or two afterwards; the pus should be cultured.

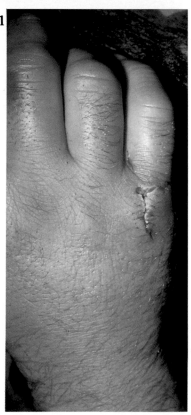

251 This man wounded his hand on another man's teeth during a fight but, if it was suspected, penetration of the joint went unrecognised and the wound was stitched up, with disastrous consequences.

Comment (i) Human teeth are more dangerous than other animals' as a source of infection.
(ii) Such a wound should be explored with the fist closed, as it was when the wound was inflicted. With the hand flat on the table, wounds in the skin, tendon and the capsule of the joint may not coincide, with the result that the penetration of the joint can go unrecognised. Military surgeons have long been aware of the fact that the straight track made by a missile or a weapon is likely to become broken up as the separate layers alter their relative positions when the wounded person changes posture. As far as possible, therefore, a penetrating wound should be explored with the part in the position in which it was injured.

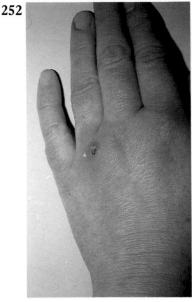

252 In spite of the benign appearance, beta-haemolytic streptococci were grown from this sore on a butcher's knuckle.

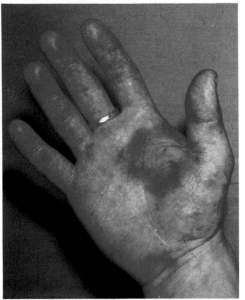

253 Erysipeloid. The red swelling caused no more than a slightly stiff feeling and was neither hot nor tender. The patient was a poulterer and had contracted erysipeloid.

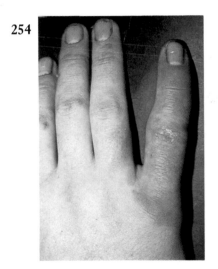

254 A more typical example of erysipeloid, which may spread down one finger and up the next. The edge of the redness is well defined and slightly raised but the colour is usually slightly duller than shown in these photographs.

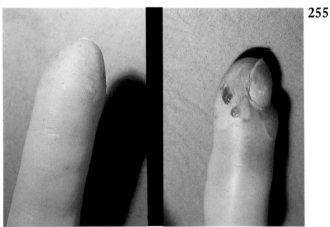

255 Herpetic whitlow is rare but is most often seen in nurses looking after tracheostomes. At first the finger is swollen, tender and dispro-portionately painful. It is liable to be incised but, if it escapes this error, after a day or two vesicles appear and then dry up as scabs, in the more familiar but less painful succession of 'cold spots' on the lips.

256 The typical appearance of deep-seated infection of the thumb that should have been explored some time before. The soft, pouting granulations with thin pus exuding from them have been likened, in crude but memorable terms, to a duck's vent. There were others on the dorsum. Six weeks before, an open fracture-dislocation had been repaired with the aid of a Kirschner's wire and for most of the time since had been recorded variously as, 'healing slowly'; 'granulating nicely'; 'not quite healed', etc. The site was subjected to numerous changes of dressing and antibiotics—and even to silver nitrate.

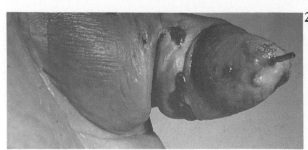

Comment If a wound has not healed or nearly so in about 3 weeks, there may well be a surgically remediable cause such as infection or foreign matter. In this case, the wound was healed, without the use of antibiotics, a fortnight after removing what was left of the tip of the thumb and applying a split skin graft to the raw surface as soon as the bleeding had stopped.

Swelling and deformity

Important as the history of the injury may be, it can be misleading, with the result that the patient or the doctor underestimates the damage that has been caused. As mentioned earlier, pain and swelling after injury of a finger call for radiological as well as clinical examination.

257

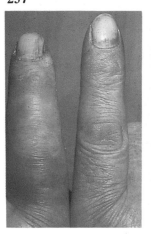

258

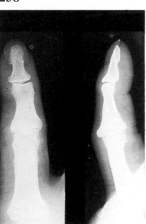

259

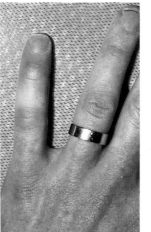

260

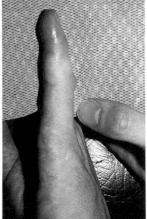

257 and 258 The patient sought advice because after a fortnight the finger that he thought he had bruised at work was still troubling him.

The fact that he had continued to use it may have done more good than harm.

259 and 260 In spite of the normal appearance, the tip of the finger had been dislocated.

Comment As well as being xrayed, the painful, swollen finger should be examined for abnormal movement by the 'wobble test'.

261 and 262 The external deformity of the thumb was less than one might expect with interphalangeal dislocation.

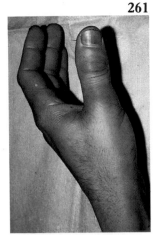

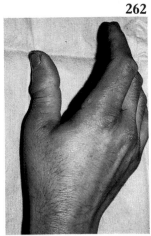

263 and 264 This injury was 2 months old. The patient accepted the advice that any treatment at that stage would interfere with the use of his thumb.

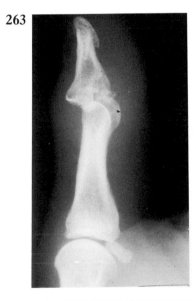

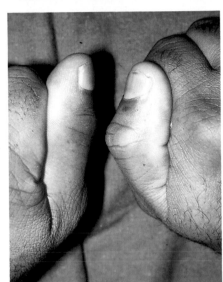

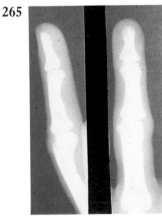

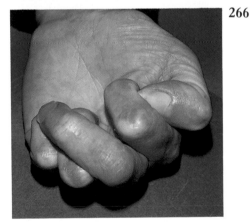

265 and 266 In this case the fracture looked mild. The shape of the finger suggested that it required no more than protection but when it was bent (**266**), it was obvious that the bone had been twisted at the fracture.

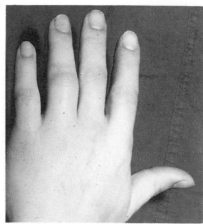

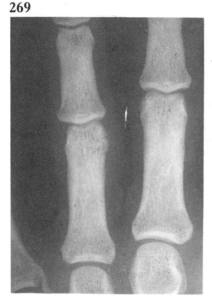

267 Injured fingers. This man complained of pain and swelling in his ring finger after being kicked while playing rugby football.

268 This degree of deformity (under anaesthesia) is not necessary to show that the joint is unstable—'wobbles'.

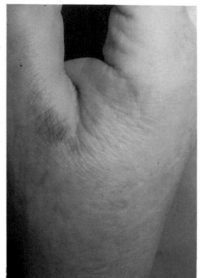

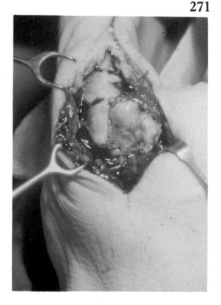

269 Xrays revealed a fairly large and quite unexpected avulsion fracture at the base of the little finger. The man had not complained of this finger but a second look at **268** suggests that excessive abduction at the base of the finger was possible. Careful examination of the xray film identified slight asymmetry of the proximal interphalangeal joint of the ring finger; exploration confirmed the possibility that this was because the capsule had been trapped in the joint. This does not happen always.

270 and 271 Wrenching injuries of the thumb can tear the ulnar collateral ligament of the metacarpophalangeal joint. In this case there was visible bruising but this does not occur always. The wobble test can be carried out, carefully, without anaesthesia.

When explored, the lesion is obvious when the thumb is out of joint but when the incision is made the torn ligament may be hidden by the extensor hood; repeat the wobble test at this stage.

Comment The extensor hood and tendon lie close to the two double hooks; the head of the metacarpal lies immediately to the right of the tendon, with the stump of the collateral ligament next to the Langenbeck's retractor.

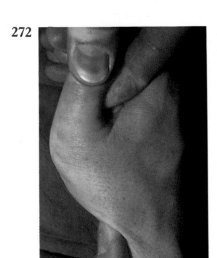

272

273

272 Rupture of the radial collateral ligament is much rarer.
Carpometacarpal injuries. These are rare and are easily overlooked.

273 This swelling, which was mainly on the ulnar side, obviously needed xray examination.

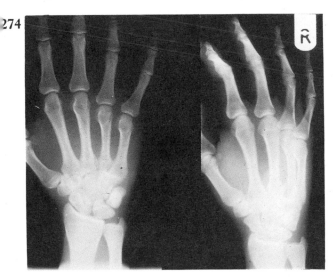

274

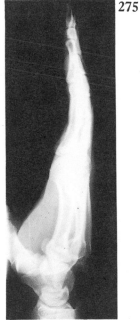

275

274 The usual anteroposterior and oblique views might be passed as normal by a young emergency room officer.

Comment Radiographers often provide oblique rather than lateral views of the hands (and also the feet), so that the shadows of the metacarpal bones are not superimposed. This makes for clarity but it can mask deformities. When fracture is suspected, therefore, lateral views of the bones or joints under suspicion must be requested, the overlapping shadows examined with care and any further advice sought immediately from experienced sources.

275 The lateral view showed clearly the fracture-dislocation of at least the 5th carpometacarpal joint. Returning to the anteroposterior view in **274**, one can see that whereas there are spaces visible at the 2nd and 3rd carpometacarpal joints, there are none at the 4th and 5th.

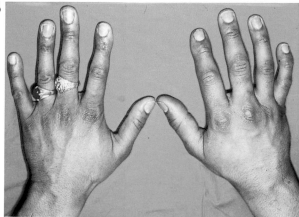

276 At first sight, the right hand might not excite much comment but the little finger appeared to be hyperextended at its base.

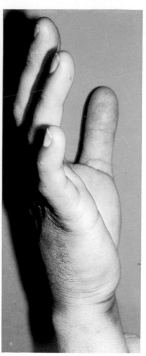

277 This was confirmed by looking from another direction.

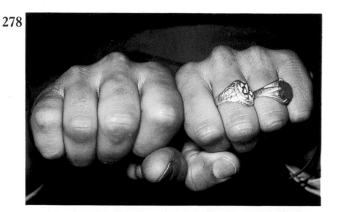

278 When the fist was closed, it could be seen that the head of the 5th metacarpal had dropped. There was dorsal tenderness at the base of this bone.

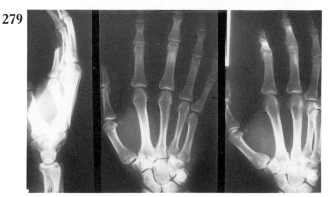

279 Careful examination of the three different xray views showed that the 5th metacarpal had **tilted forwards** at its far end and had been displaced backwards on the hamate bone.

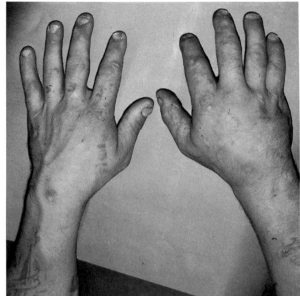

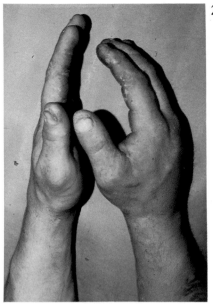

280 The right hand was injured in a motor-cycle accident. It was generally swollen and it looked broader and shorter than the left.

281 The fingers could not be straightened any further than shown.

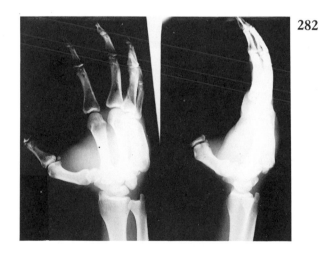

282 Xrays showed dislocation of 4 of the 5 carpometacarpal joints.

282 Xrays showed dislocation of 4 of the 5 carpometacarpal joints.

Comment Because carpometacarpal injuries are rare they may not come to mind. In the last case the history suggested that the right hand had been gripping the handlebar when the cycle crashed and that the four metacarpal bones had been driven off the carpus by the force of the impact. The hand looked broad because of the swelling and because the metacarpus had been shortened. The displaced metacarpals' bases had interfered with the action of the extensor muscles.

To the discerning ear and eye this injury is readily suspected on clinical grounds and confidently confirmed with the aid of xrays. Unless the bones are replaced (they usually require internal fixation to prevent redisplacement), the hand is permanently crippled.

Bennett's fracture-subluxation is not a frequent injury. After the first few hours it is easy to assume that swelling and tenderness are present in the anatomical snuffbox and to concentrate radiological attention on the scaphoid bone. Within the first hour or two after the injury, which is usually an ill-delivered punch rather than a fall on to the hand, the swelling is definitely distal to the snuffbox.

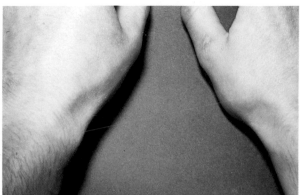

283 Bennett's injury of the right thumb. It is the hump and not the hollow that is tender. With care, it may be possible to demonstrate that pulling on the thumb abolishes the hump and that pushing it restores it (the so-called telescoping movement).

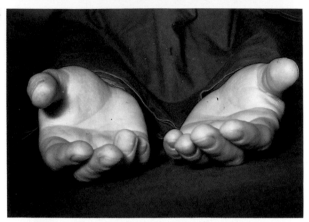

284 Another characteristic feature of this injury is the fact that the thenar eminence is swollen; this is not obliterated by the passage of time. Rarely, Bennett's injury causes visible bruising in the palm.

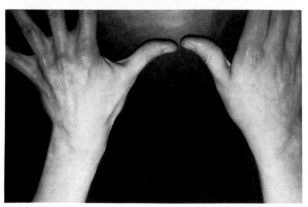

285 This man had been using his thumb since injuring it a week before.

286 and 287 It is questionable whether there is any advantage in treating Bennett's fracture (and disabling the patient) at this stage. Note that the thenar eminence was still swollen. Some weeks later the patient expressed satisfaction with the thumb.

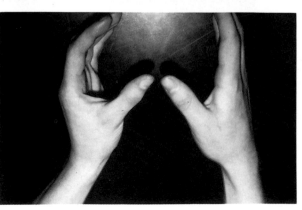

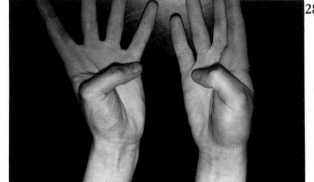

288-290 Even 10 years after Bennett's injury the function can be much better than the xray appearance. The right thumb had been injured.

Comment It can be asked reasonably if it is justifiable to disable a person by treating a condition that is no more than an inconvenience and is not likely to become worse.

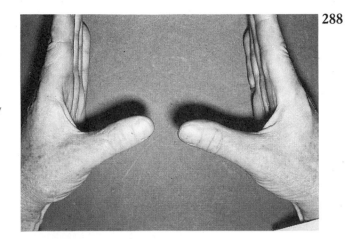

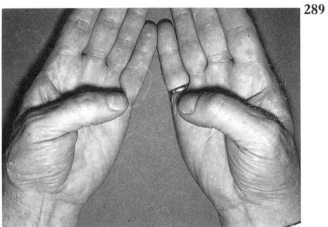

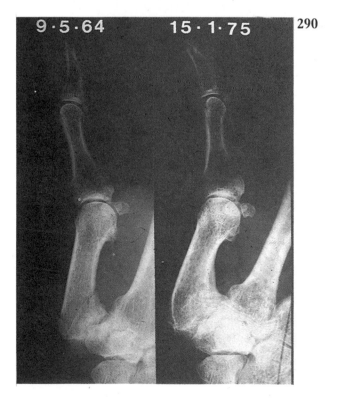

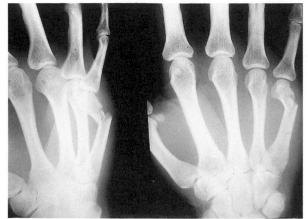

291 This hand had been injured by a punch 2 weeks before but had been used ever since.

292

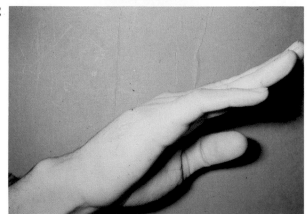

292 and 293 The loss of movement at the base of the little finger is perhaps less surprising than the lack of external deformity.

In many cases deformities are obvious rather than subtle; some require special treatment and some require none.

293

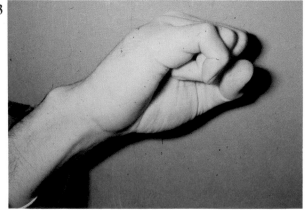

294 Manipulation did not correct this metacarpo-phalangeal dislocation.

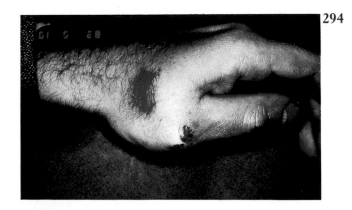

294

295 Exploration showed that the extensor tendon was trapped between the bones and that the head of the metacarpal had been blanching the skin. The tendon lies obliquely almost half-way between the blades of the retractor and the head of the metacarpal partly overlaps its lower half. After the tendon had been released the joint was easily replaced.

Comment Irreducibility by manipulation is often attributed to so-called button-holing of the capsule but this is not usually an accurate description.

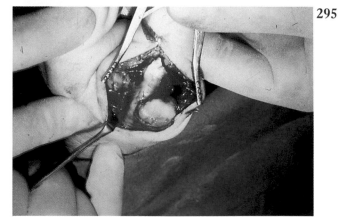

295

Posture

296 Apart from deformity, alterations in the posture of a part may be of great diagnostic value. A drooping tip and sagging middle of a finger can occur if the joints are hyperextensible. When the proximal interphalangeal joint is hyperextended, the flexor digiti profundus is effectively shortened and the fingertip is held flexed. This posture can also occur with severe mallet finger, because the extensor tendon is completely detached from the terminal phalanx and extensor power is concentrated at the lax interphalangeal joint proximal to it. This degree of mallet finger should be considered for operation while the deformity is still fully correctable and the extensor tendon can be returned to the terminal phalanx and remains of a consistency to hold stitches.

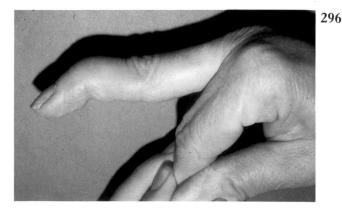

296

297

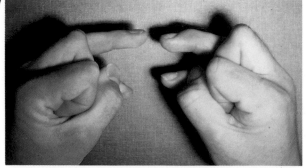

298

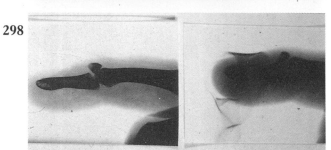

297 and 298 The right finger might be described as a mallet finger. The fracture shown in **298** might be described as a mallet finger fracture. In fact, the fingertip retained good power of extension. In the right film it is suspending quite a heavy weight.

Comment The term 'mallet finger' is correctly applied to a finger that droops at the tip (it is also known as drop finger) and this is most often the result of separation of the extensor tendon from the terminal phalanx by closed rupture or by accidental cutting. Avulsion may remove a small piece of bone from the base of the terminal phalanx; this is often referred to as a mallet finger fracture. This can be misleading in that a diagnosis of 'mallet finger fracture' implies that the treatment should be for a mallet finger.

If one looks carefully at **297** it will be seen that the fingertip is not drooping, although the swelling at the base of the nail may make it appear as though it is. In **298** the fragment is shown to be much bigger than one caused by avulsion. The explanation is that this sort of injury is caused by a combination of longitudinal compression and hyperextension that shears off the extensor lip of the terminal phalanx in continuity with the extensor tendon. It is not as well

known as it deserves to be that the extensor tendon is not attached to the edge of the terminal phalanx but extensively to its dorsal surface. As a result, it can be stripped from this surface, with a piece of bone, without becoming completely detached and so losing its ability to extend the fingertip.

If this type of injury is splinted in even slight hyperextension, this is liable to result in increased separation of the fragment and subluxation of the joint, because the original deformity is being reproduced, as is shown clearly.

It is evident that the terms 'mallet finger'; and 'mallet finger fracture' can be misapplied, with unfortunate results. Mallet finger or drop finger should be reserved for fingers with the corresponding deformity and the term mallet (finger) fracture should be abandoned in favour of mallet finger with fracture, recognising that not all bony fragments in this part have been pulled off.

299 Rupture of the middle slip of the extensor tendon is not easy to diagnose before the deformity becomes difficult to treat. This posture might be the result of an effusion into the joint and until the lateral bands become fixed at the side of the joint, active extension remains possible. It is very unusual for avulsion fractures to occur with this injury but when they are recognised they should bring it to mind; all too often the deformity is already established when the patient is first seen at hospital.

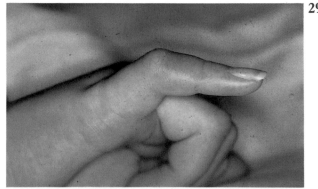

300 Rupture of the tendon of extensor pollicis longus may be caused by a degenerative condition, such as rheumatoid disease, or it can take place a few weeks after a very mild fracture affecting the dorsum of the radius in the bed of the tendon. The condition is easily diagnosed if it is in mind but it is not a frequent occurrence; the patient's complaints are often vague, such as that the thumb seems funny or that there is difficulty in gripping and twisting things.

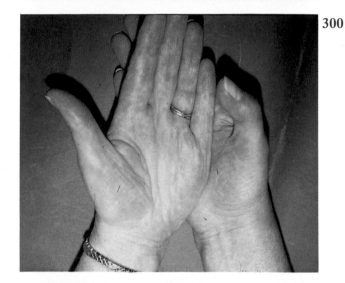

301 Delayed rupture of the tendon can also follow a wound such as the one shown here. The explanation is that the tendon was partly divided at the time of wounding but that this went undetected (and perhaps unsuspected), until rupture occurred during later use.

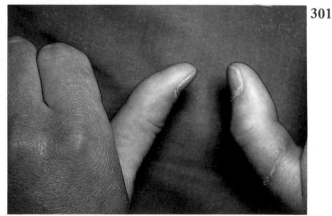

Comment When there is a cut over a tendon, the wound should be explored with the tendon in mind. When a tendon is visible in a wound, it should be watched carefully while it is put through its full range of movement. Unless the part is explored in the position in which it was wounded, a cut in a tendon may have moved out of sight.

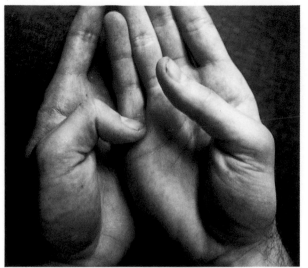

302 Rupture of extensor pollicis brevis is very rare. Note that the interphalangeal but not the metacarpophalangeal joint of the right thumb is extended. In the case of the left thumb the patient could extend the metacarpophalangeal joint while the tip was flexed.

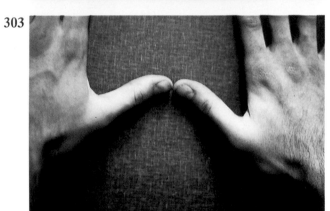

303 It can be seen that the right metacarpophalangeal joint was not fully extended with the others. Although the tendon of the right extensor pollicis brevis can be seen, it was not acting on the proximal phalanx.

Dislocation of extensor tendons

This condition most often results from attentuation and rupture caused by rheumatoid disease but it can also follow a blow that ruptures the extensor hood.

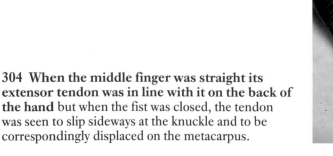

304

304 When the middle finger was straight its extensor tendon was in line with it on the back of the hand but when the fist was closed, the tendon was seen to slip sideways at the knuckle and to be correspondingly displaced on the metacarpus.

305 The tear is easily seen here and was repaired in this (another) case.

Comment A dorsal longitudinal incision gives the best exposure and causes no trouble later.

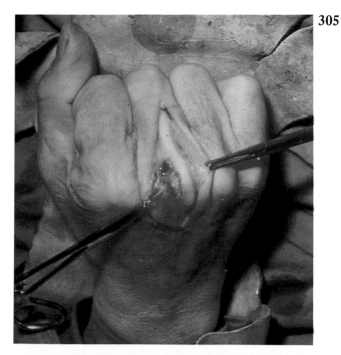

306 In a child, one of the causes of a straight forefinger is a supracondylar fracture of the humerus that has damaged the median nerve. This patient was an adult who had noticed that his right hand had become clumsy. There was no history of injury or illness, no pain and no alteration of sensibility. Flexion of both the thumb and the forefinger was much weakened.

Comment Lesions of the anterior interosseous nerve are rare; they weaken flexor pollicis longus and flexor digiti profundus of the forefinger and can be caused by fibrous bands in muscles near the origin of the nerve.

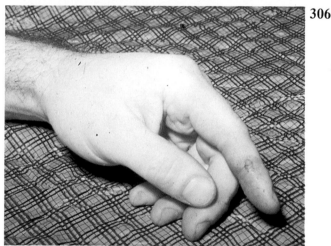

Miscellaneous conditions

Wasting

Weakness and wasting of the intrinsic muscles of the hand follow damage to the median or ulnar nerves anywhere from the wrist upwards.

307 Wasting of the 1st dorsal interosseous muscle is perhaps the most sensitive visible evidence of an ulnar nerve lesion or of its deep branch in the palm (*see* **243**).

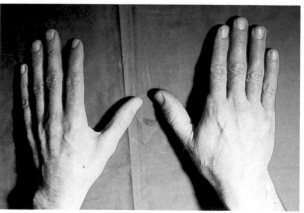

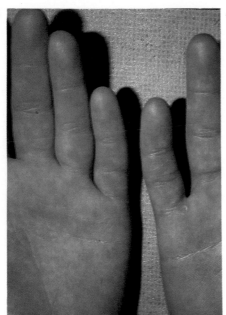

308 With lesions at or above the wrist there is also wasting of the little finger but it takes a week or two to appear.

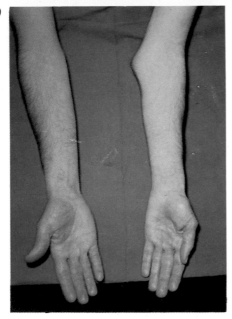

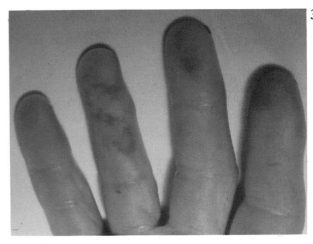

309 With lesions at or above the elbow, wasting of the ulnar side of the forearm is present as well. There are also weakness, numbness and tingling in the distribution of the nerve. This was a case of delayed ulnar palsy following malunion of a fracture of the capitulum.

310 Sensitivity to cold. Ever since it had been crushed, this man's ring finger had been unduly sensitive to cold, which made it look blotchy rather than generally pale. The explanation was thought to be that the main arteries had been crushed.

Dressings and slings

These are inseparable from the treatment of most injuries of the hands, but they do not always receive the attention that they deserve. Dressings support; they protect both mechanically and against bacterial invasion; they absorb discharge and they hide what is objectionable or unsightly. The last function is the least easily justified, especially if the use of the part is thereby impeded or completely prevented.

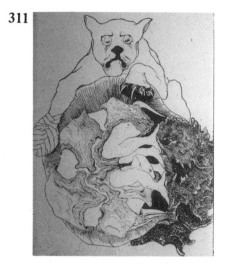

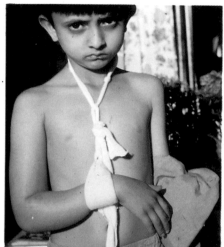

311 This illustration had been taken from Kipling's 'Just So Story' about the beginning of the armadillos, in which a young jaguar sustained multiple pricks of one paw. It shows the neat spica pattern of the bandage and it illustrates three frequent causes of trouble. These are damage, disuse and dependency, which will each cause swelling and in combination they can be disastrous. The swelling caused by injury is preventable by firm bandaging and elevation; the disuse may be inevitable for a time but there is no excuse for swelling caused by dependency. This can occur in the absence of any injury of the hand.

312 Swelling of the hand. A collar and cuff sling used for a mild supracondylar fracture of the humerus caused disuse, dependency and swelling of an uninjured hand.

Comment If the hand requires a dressing that renders it temporarily unusable, the fingers should be bent at right angles at the metacarpophalangeal joints but otherwise kept straight and the thumb should also be straight and abducted from the palm. This has sometimes been referred to as the 'writing position' but the most fitting term is the 'position for splintage'; it is the position from which recovering movement is least difficult if the hand becomes stiff. The term 'position of function' has been used but the hand has so many functions that the term is meaningless.

In the interest of function, dressings should be as small as is consistent with their purpose in any particular case. They should also be snug, tidy and removed when they have served their purpose. The all-too-popular fingerstall is often a sign of lack of confidence and becomes a cause of disuse and even stiffness. If its use is permitted, these complications must be guarded against.

The earliest return to work is good for morale and it is often the best form of physiotherapy, not least because the patient gets paid for it. It is not always appreciated, particularly by junior doctors, that seeing that the patient returns to work as soon as possible is as much their responsibility as was the insertion of stitches or other surgical measures. A suitable representative of the employer should be contacted, so as to try and ensure that the patient does go back to therapeutic activity and is not allowed to idle about, not using the hand. The head of the firm or the personnel manager, not the foreman, is the person to approach for this purpose. It is a wise rule not to discharge the patient from hospital until he or she is ready to return to work.

6 Hip to leg

Bruises and grazes

Hip and thigh

Extensive bruises result in considerable loss of blood from circulation but the loss is not usually so fast as to produce obvious changes in colour, pulse rate or blood pressure.

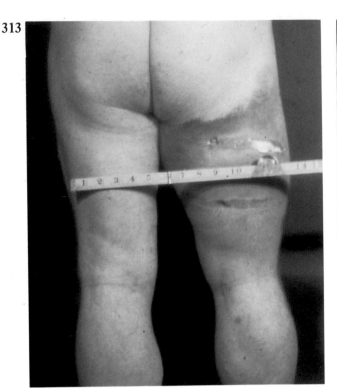

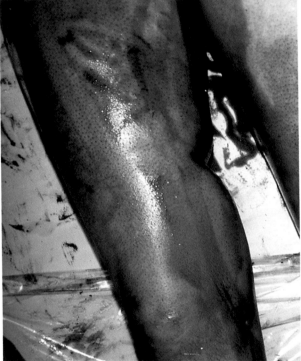

313 Extensive bruising. The right thigh is at least 1 inch bigger in diameter which represents an increase in volume of between 2 and 3 litres of blood.

Comment When a large haematoma in a layer of fat liquefies, it becomes a large floppy swelling that feels rather like a partly filled rubber hot-water bottle attached to the part that is affected. Whether before or after liquefaction, a haematoma cannot be completely evacuated except by laying it widely open, after which suction drainage is necessary for several days until the raw surfaces of the cleft have stuck together.

314 A tractor turned over and a projection on it was responsible for the dent seen in the right thigh. (The discoloration was caused by oil.) When the dent was palpated, it was obvious that the skin had been depressed almost as far as the femur, with crushing of the intervening fat and muscles. The result can fairly be called a soft-centred bruise and is of considerable diagnostic value. Following repair, the skin was for some time tethered by the underlying scar.

Knee and leg

315 Massive bruising of the thigh and leg that was caused when an old man was struck by a vehicle coming from his left. The bruise was felt to have a soft centre on each side. On the right, the thumb had only skin between it and the tibia; on the left, the fingertip was separated from the medial condyle of the femur by no more than skin. Exploration confirmed that the extensor muscles had been crushed through (and the anterior tibial artery severed) and that the medial ligament of the knee had been torn from the femur.

Comment A bruise should always be felt, because this may provide useful evidence of the degree of underlying damage.

316 Extensive bruising accompanying a mild-looking fracture of the fibula. The skin had just begun to blister. In an adult, this amount of swelling of the leg represents the loss of more than a litre of blood into it.

Comment (i) Blisters over a large and superficial bruise suggest that the skin is being dangerously overstretched and that the haematoma should be evacuated to relieve it.
(ii) Divergence of the upper fragment of the fibula from the tibia suggested that the muscles between them had been torn. Occasionally, the anterior tibial artery is torn as well and ischaemic necrosis of the extensor muscles follows. In this case, the artery had not been damaged.

317 With a superficial bruise like this under old skin, breakdown is inevitable but the skin lost was less than half the width and length of the area outlined.

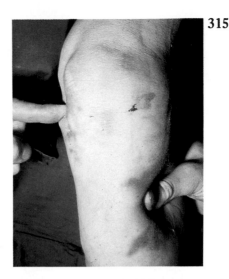

315

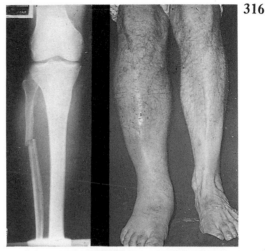

316

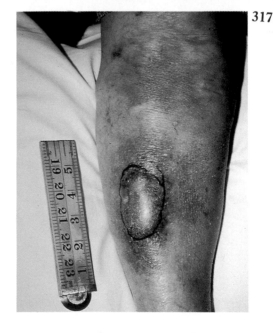

317

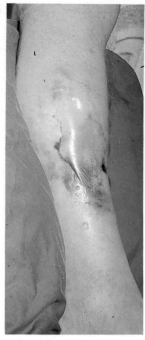

318 The skin did not survive this blistering, which was the result of local damage rather than tense swelling.

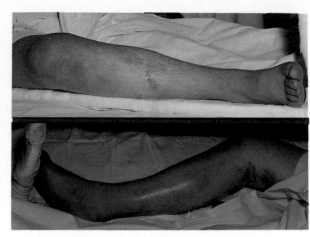

319 The marked swelling that accompanied fracture of the tibia and fibula was obvious, as was the dusky appearance of the foot. The front of the shin shows the mark of impact (in a motor-cycle accident) that broke the tibia. The blood stains came from a small wound on the back of the calf, which had been caused by puncture from within. Exploration confirmed that much of the calf muscle and the posterior tibial artery had been torn through by the tibia. In spite of having a large amount of torn muscle removed from his calf, the youth was able to resume playing badminton several months later, after the fracture had healed soundly (*see* also **230**).

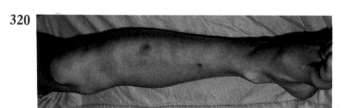

320 A boy struck his left leg while tobogganing. His 2 pairs of wet and closely fitting trousers were removed with some difficulty but without complaint from the boy. This made fracture seem unlikely but the small bruise on the shin had a soft centre and there was a fracture of the tibia under it.

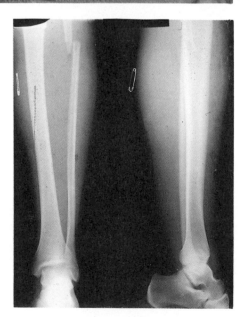

321 A motor-cyclist was struck on the left leg by a car. There was a small wound near the fracture of the fibula. However, the most important feature of the xray was the presence of the subcutaneous air bubbles well below the middle of the leg.

322 Because of the presence of air bubbles, the leg was explored and a large amount of pulped extensor muscle was found and removed. The belly of tibialis anterior and its tendon remained in continuity. The incision was necessarily long; some of the marks of impact are visible just beyond the incision. There were some more obvious marks of impact in front.

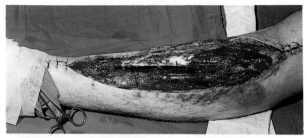

323 The left and middle panels show comminution of the fibula and air bubbles nearby. The notes stated that the victim, who was a pedal cyclist, had been struck by a passing motor vehicle; they also stated that there had been brisk bleeding and that the wound had been explored, though no details of exploration were given. The wound had been closed. The right panel shows the fine, diffused bubbles of gas gangrene that developed within 24 hours. The man lost his leg but not his life.

Comment In spite of the clear record of evidence that there had been a forcible impact and that the anterior tibial artery might have been torn, it seemed that the wound had been explored with a finger rather than the eye. It had not been noted whether or not the trousers had been torn. If clothing has been torn over a wound caused by a heavy blow, it is possible that some material has been driven into the wound.

324 When the damaged area is small it may seem prudent to make any necessary incision through undamaged skin, as in this case. The fact that skin between the incision and the original (circular) damaged area died may be because any remaining blood supply was cut off by the incision. If this was so, it suggests that if an incision has to be made it should, whenever practicable, be through the damaged part, where it would add less damage than if it were made through undamaged tissue.

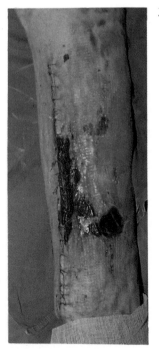

Comment After adopting this policy, the author had no cause to regret it in about 20 years.

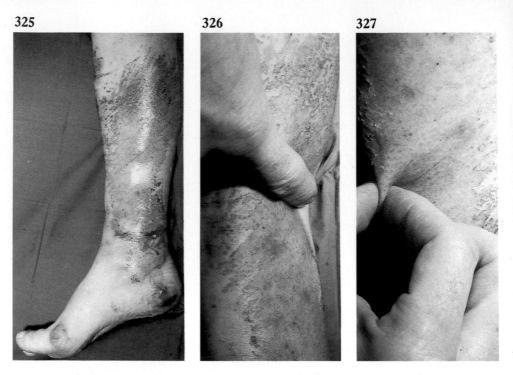

325 **326** **327**

325 The appearance of a woman's leg that had been run over by a milk van. The skin had not been broken but it had been badly grazed and crushed.

326 and 327 It was obvious to the fingers that it had been stripped extensively from the underlying fat. Ten days later, most of the damaged skin had died.

Comment From time to time it is necessary to make a cut in skin that has been damaged. When the damage is as extensive as it was in the last case, any cut that has to be made can only be through damaged skin.

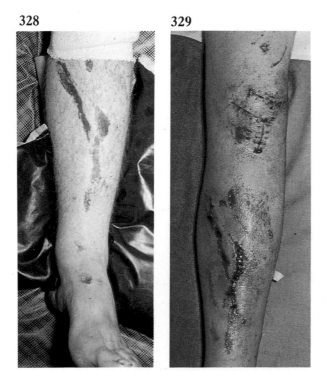

328 **329**

328 and 329 If the skin that is cut is already dead or doomed, it will at least be held together by stitches and they will close the wound until the extent of excision and grafting has become clear.

330 At first sight this wound of the shin might be taken for a puncture by the broken tibia beneath it. However, on close examination it was obvious that the graze had been caused by heavy pressure. Under anaesthesia it was found that the fat beneath the graze over the shin had been split. This can often be recognised by the use of a probe or other fairly fine instrument of adequate length but if the wound is large enough to admit a finger, this is even better. The dent can also be felt from the outside. If this skin had to be cut, the cut would have been made through the split in the fat. In this case the skin was protected from risk of harmful pressure by displacement of the fracture in plaster by the use of external skeletal fixation and it healed uneventfully. As a general rule, wounds accompanying fractures should not be closed until the fracture has been manipulated.

Comment Puncture wounds are most often made from within and they usually heal well if they are merely dressed; excision enlarges the wound and makes it more difficult to close. If there is a large haematoma, a puncture wound may be used to insert a suction drain. Whether they are caused from within or from without, wounds larger than a puncture should be explored because they may contain foreign matter or dirt on bone that had come out and gone back again.

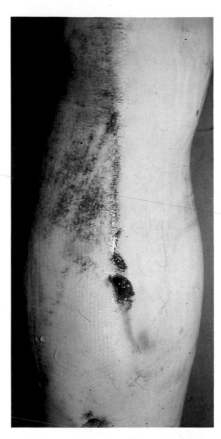

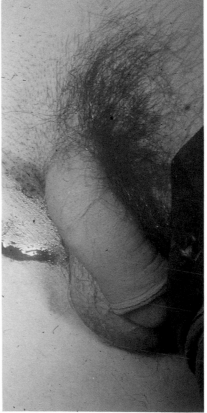

Wounds

Hip and thigh

331 When they are boning meat, butchers sometimes stab themselves accidentally in the groin. This wound bled little, there were normal pulses beyond and there was no evidence of damage to the femoral nerve. It was judged to be suitable for closure with local analgesia and the stitch marks can be seen. Fortunately, a shrewd registrar with military surgical experience came to know about this and at once arranged for the wound to be explored carefully under general anaesthesia. A finger may be informative in identifying the direction if not the depth of a wound but it should be used only when the operation is ready to start. The 10-inch incision that was made gave comfortable access to the femoral vessels above and below, so that they could be occluded at once if serious bleeding began. The artery was undamaged but a wound in the vein, which had been sealed (and might have healed itself spontaneously), was found and repaired.

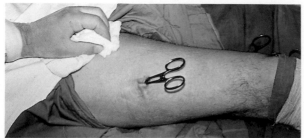

332 Another accidental stab wound in the thigh. The forceps gave wrong information about the direction of the wound; as the nature of the accident suggested, the track was almost perpendicular to the surface.

Comment When a finger can be placed in a wound (*see* 88), it is more informative than a metal tool and is less likely to make a false passage. Anything that is used as a probe, which is still a very useful tool, should be held gently between finger and thumb and not firmly in the fist; it should be used as though it were a cat's whisker, not a poker.

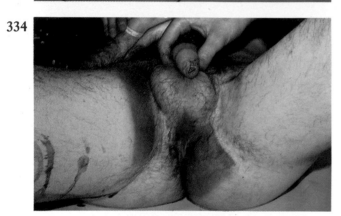

333 This man was shot in the thigh while he was sitting in his car.

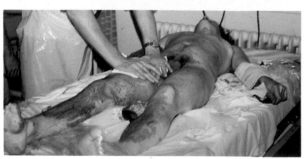

334 There was extensive bruising in the perineum and blood in the urethra because the (low velocity) bullet had passed up the thigh, had been deflected by the pubis and severed the urethra as it passed across the pelvis. The victim made an uneventful recovery after a catheter had been passed across the gap under vision and temporary drainage of the bladder had been provided. A full-size sound has been passed easily every year or two since. The bullet was not removed and caused no trouble.

335 A close-range accidental wound by a sawn-off shotgun removed much of the front of the thigh and 6 inches of the femoral artery. It was a fine achievement of those on the spot and in the ambulance that the victim reached hospital alive. A careful search for the wads among the pulped muscle was successful. Wads are now increasingly made of plastic material which, unlike the old sort, do not carry Clostridia. Neither sort shows up on xray films.

336 At slightly longer range the pellets have begun to scatter; there was no possibility in this case that a wad had entered the thigh. In the absence of fracture, neural or vascular damage a wound with so many small punctures may be better kept under close observation than explored (*see* **136** and **202**), but antibiotics and tetanus toxoid should be given on admission to hospital.

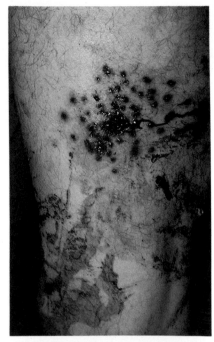

336

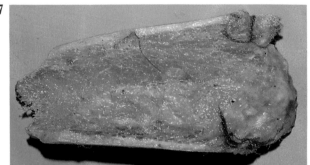

337 Sometimes large loose fragments of bone accompany the victim of severe open fractures to hospital. They can be cleaned, boiled and replaced in the interest of restoring stability to the broken bone.

338 The fragment (shown in 337) adjoins the lower part of the blade-plate.

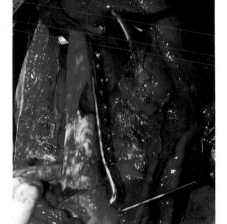

338

Comment Bone is no more dead for having been boiled than for being thrown out of the body in the first place, indeed it is the only certainly dead tissue that it is legitimate either to leave or to replace in the body. However, this procedure should not be undertaken unless the wound is fresh and the standard of the surgical toilet is high. Incorporation of the dead bone and its revival take many months. This patient was able to walk without crutches or sticks 18 months after his accident.

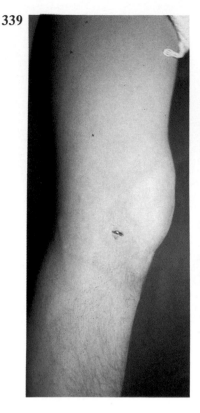

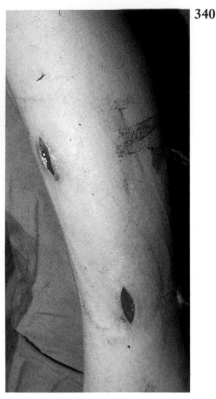

339 A puncture wound near a joint may enter it.
There was a small effusion into this joint. Sometimes synovial liquid comes out or air goes in. Therefore, the joint should be xrayed.

Small wounds can admit unexpected foreign bodies.

340 A small wound on the leg after a fall. By the time this photograph was taken the leg had become infected and on draining the abscess a splinter about 4 inches long was removed.

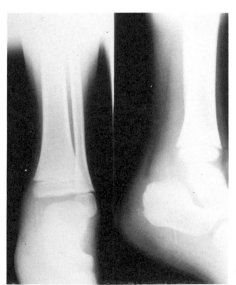

341 A small wound on the heel had given entry to a short piece of pencil, which is just visible on the xray film.

Comment The history may include little or nothing to suggest the presence of a foreign body and not all those that are suspected are easily recognisable, or indeed demonstrable, with xrays. When a foreign body that might be present is not visible on xray films, it is better not to explore a small wound such as a puncture. A long and fruitless search can do a great deal of damage when it is carried out with determination or desperation rather than discretion. Such a wound should be presumed to be contaminated with bacteria and should be treated with an antibiotic and rest. If a foreign body is present, it is easily dealt with if an abscess forms and has to be drained.

342 Fracture with external wound. This patient's considerate attitude was suitably rewarded. She fell on the stairs at home, dragged herself to bed and did not want to bother her doctor until after the weekend. For nearly 48 hours, the only dressing for the wound was a grubby blanket. There was extensive bruising. The fracture was not severe and it was decided to leave it to nature by cleansing the limb, dressing the wound and applying a plaster cast with a window over the wound. Within 3 weeks the wound had healed; the fracture followed suit some weeks later.

Comment It is not true that bones are filled with black ingratitude, but it would be unwise to rely on the prophylactic properties of a grubby blanket.

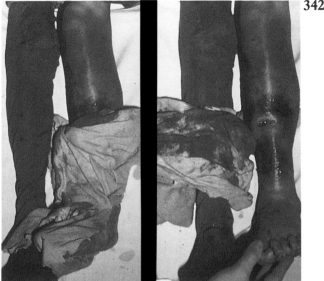

343 Large wounds may be the result of retraction of the skin and distortion of the limb; if so, they can be closed quite easily by simple suture, but secure fixation of the underlying fractures may be necessary to protect the suture line.

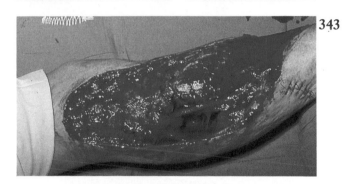

344 The above wound of the lower limb healed uneventfully after internal fixation and suture.

Comment Delayed primary suture should be considered in such cases; if a fracture is plated, exposure of a plate for a few days is not of itself detrimental to healing.

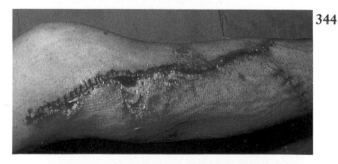

345 A large and destructive wound that was caused when a bus ran over a girl's leg. Much crushed muscle had to be removed but no skin had been lost and the wound was sewn up.

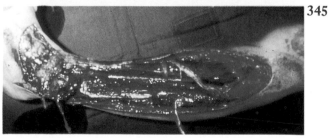

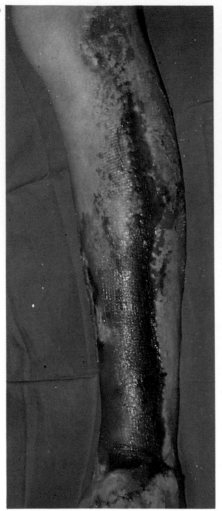

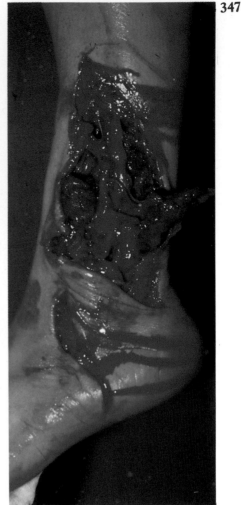

346 Nearly 3 weeks later the amount of dead skin that had to be removed was clearly visible. There was no infection and split skin grafts were applied at once to the healthy, raw surface beneath the dead skin. The skin grafts took well.

347 In spite of their appearance and an underlying fracture, these wounds healed well after surgical toilet, internal fixation and suture.

Comment In the last two cases it should be noted how close the stitches in the main wound were to each other and to the edge of the skin. They were of 3/0 size. It is a mistake to take large bites with strong material, because this not only concentrates the tension in the skin at a few points but increases it unnecessarily. This is because the skin within the bite is not stretched and its edges can be brought together only by overstretching the rest. If fine, closely set stitches are used, they distribute the tension more widely and make use of all the skin that is available to come together. It may be argued that so many stitches so close together and so close to the edge of the wound will kill the edge. This may be so, but the edges remain together and the wound remains sealed. It takes longer to heal and the stitches should be left for 3 or even 4 weeks. The stitches should be inserted from the ends to the middle of the wound, so that each bears only a little more tension than the one before. This method takes time but it is time well spent.

Infection

Any wound can become infected, whatever its origins. The external appearance of a wound does not always correspond with what is going on beneath the surface (*see* **58** and **256**).

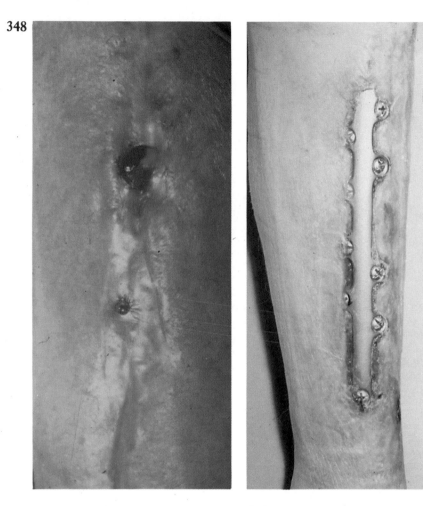

348 Even one small sinus with pouting granulations over implanted metal means that there is infection, which can be very extensive, although perhaps no more than skin deep. Medicaments applied to the surface are useless; in due course the metal must be removed.

349 This extent of exposure is unusual, as is the absence of discharge. The man walked about for weeks with only a light dressing while the fracture mended. Removing the plate was then very easy.

Swelling and deformity

Hip and thigh

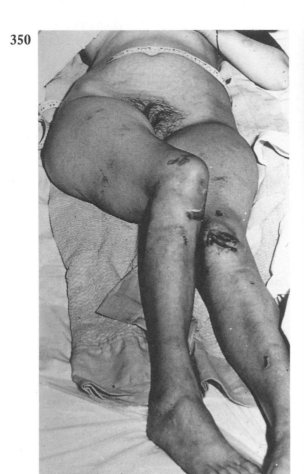

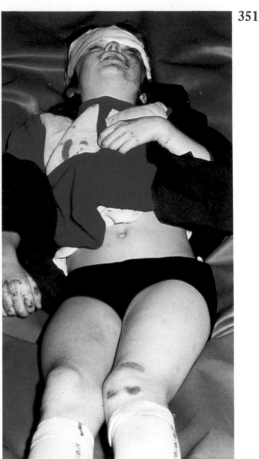

350 The typical appearance of posterior dislocation of the hip; the wounds on the knees were made by the dashboard of a crashing car and the impact drove the right hip out of joint. Adduction, flexion and medial rotation of the limb are well shown.

351 Dislocation of the left hip was rightly suspected but it was not confirmed—a safe mistake.

Comment (i) Dislocation of the hip can be overlooked easily when there is also a fracture of the shaft of the femur because the fracture is the obvious cause of the swelling and shortening and its presence prevents the limb from adopting the familiar position of flexion, adduction and medial rotation. The combination is rare but it should be thought of after a high-speed crash. Also remember that when there is wide separation at a fracture of the shaft of the femur, this may be because the proximal fragment has been

flexed and adducted by dislocation of the hip. The knowing eye will look for this sign and insist that the hip joint be xrayed. The knowing hand may detect the prominence of the greater trochanter.
(ii) Fracture-dislocation of the hip does not cause the limb to adopt the typical posture, because the hip joint remains movable. In a fat or unconscious person or when there is a fracture elsewhere in the limb, fracture-dislocation of the hip can be overlooked easily, unless it is thought of and the hip is xrayed.

352 This posture is characteristic of anterior dislocation of the hip. The mark on the knee is the site of the impact that dislocated the hip by excessive abduction.

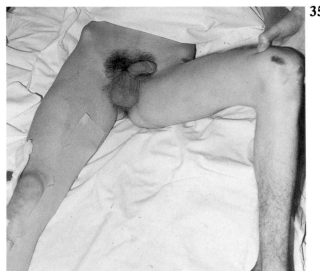

353 This man had his hip forced into such a wide abduction that it was dislocated forwards; his account of the accident was both clear and informative. The limb lay in a more natural resting posture than in the previous case but the leg and foot were swollen and dusky.

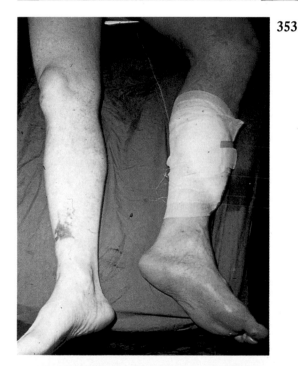

354 There was a prominence in the groin, where a hard lump could be felt. The colour of the limb returned to normal when the hip was put back in join and the pressure of the head of the femur was removed from the femoral vein. The nerve and the artery were not affected.

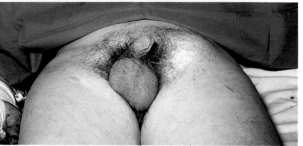

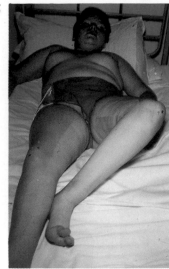

355

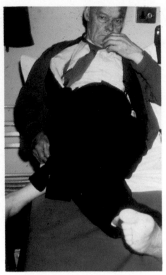

356

A tall boy, who was heavy for his age of 13 years, complained of pain in his left knee after stumbling, which might easily have twisted the knee. The left thigh looked slightly swollen and the front of the hip was tender.

355 When he flexed his hip the abnormal amount of lateral rotation that appeared was consistent with a slipped upper epiphysis of the femur, which was confirmed by xrays. The old adage, 'Pain in the knee, examine the hip', applies after injury as well as without it, especially in children.

356 The posture and apparent unconcern of a man with two fractures of the shaft of his left femur, which was draped over and comfortably supported by the right thigh. He remained unconcerned even when his trousers were removed carefully, without altering the position of the injured limb.

Comment All too often, the diagnosis of a fracture is held to require the application of splints. When this is done carefully, it supports the limb and makes it much more comfortable. However, applying splints can be a painful procedure that is of no benefit to the patient. Comfortable support is what the limb needs from the beginning; this can be provided in many unconventional ways that in a first aid competition would not be given the credit they deserved. In this case the first aid was excellent; those responsible were commended.

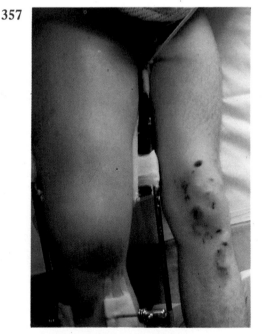

357

357 The massive swelling of this thigh far exceeded what might have been expected after a fracture that did not appear to be very serious. In fact, the femoral artery had been partly torn and the foot became ischaemic. The swelling so raised the pressure within the intact fascial envelope of the thigh as to cause Volkmann's ischaemia and intense myoglobinuria—a striking variation of the crush syndrome. The patient lost his limb but this may be the only way to save life. The decision to amputate may have to be taken so early that it is almost unthinkable.

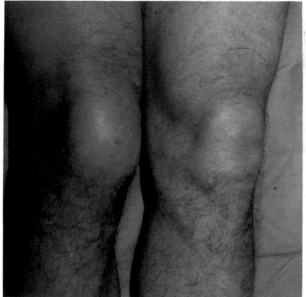

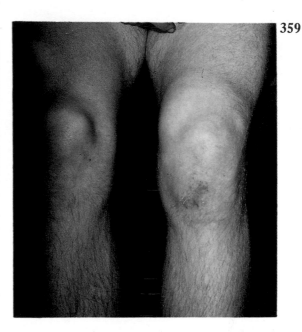

358 The accurately localised swelling caused by an enlarged prepatellar bursa.

Comment Mild fractures may not be very obvious but they should be suspected if there is a lipohae-marthrosis.

359 Well-marked swelling around the patella caused by an effusion into the knee joint. This patient walked into the hospital and was found to have a fracture of the patella. The mark of impact was well shown.

360

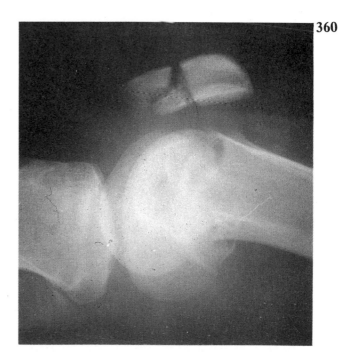

360 In this case the fractures were obvious, as was the clear distinction between fat above and blood below in the effusion as seen in a lateral view of the joint.

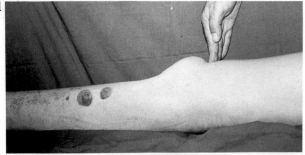

361 An elderly man missed his footing and felt something give way in his knee; he could no longer walk. The knee was not very swollen but there was an easily palpable gap where the quadriceps had been pulled off the patella.

Comment Sometimes only the rectus femoris is ruptured and this may be overlooked because the victim may still be able to hobble; active extension of the knee is still possible and, if there is a tense effusion into the joint, the gap above the patella may not be palpable.

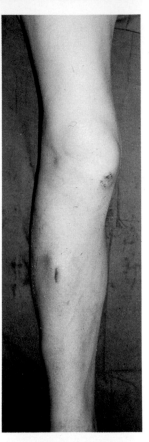

362 There was not much swelling of this knee after the patient had been knocked down in the road; the discerning eye will recognise marks of impact by the vehicle on the leg and by contact of the inner side of the knee with the road. As suspected, the medial ligament had been torn.

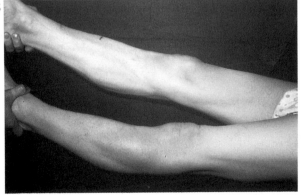

363 This left knee had been injured in a fall. The hyperextension by gravity and the lateral swelling were suggestive and stressing in adduction was conclusive of rupture of the lateral ligament.

Comment Fracture of the lateral condyle also leads to instability (when a valgus stress is applied) but the swelling is further forward and less well defined, being of deeper origin.

364 A rugby footballer complained of pain and 'something slipping', when his left knee was forcibly bent and twisted in a scrum. Thoughts of a torn meniscus were dispelled by the absence of an effusion into the joint and by the presence of the head of the fibula well forward of its normal position.

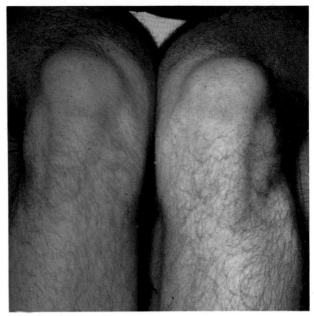

Comment The story and the findings were typical but dislocation of the head of the fibula is rare.

When the patella dislocates, its articular surface usually lies against the outer side of the lateral condyle of the femur and its transverse axis is directed fore and aft. The patient's account of what happened may be to the effect that something seemed to slip, the knee gave way and could not be straightened until somebody did something, something seemed to go back and the knee could then be moved again. The resemblance to tearing a meniscus is obvious, but an astute examiner may be aware of this and ask if, when the knee was 'locked', there was a lump. The answer may be that there was but that it was on the inner side. That is because when the patella slips to the side of the knee it leaves the medial condyle of the femur looking prominent and it was that rather than the lateral prominence that the patient saw. Recurrent subluxation of the patella may give rise to a similar story but in both cases there is tenderness on the medial edge of the patella; any attempt to test its lateral mobility evokes an apprehensive reaction by the patient. In the case of recurrent subluxation the patient is often a girl and the patella may be small; sometimes the other knee is affected as well.

365 Occasionally, the patella slips sideways without turning round the femur and it sticks out like a shelf on the outside of the knee. In this view from below the thigh is on the left.

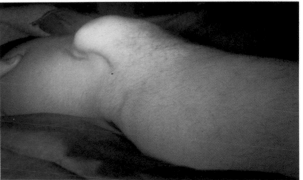

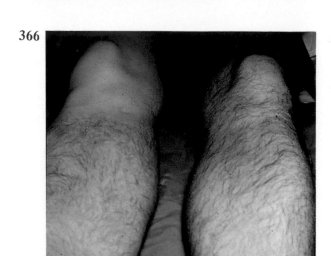

366 'Something stuck' in this man's right knee and he could not bend it. The right patella appeared to be slightly higher than the left; this was so because it had become hitched on an osteophyte at the upper margin of the articular surface of the femur.

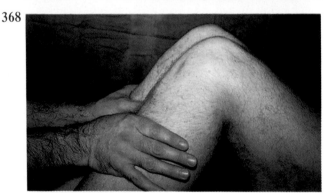

367 The knee was obviously out of shape after a heavy blow and it looked as though the leg (which is to the left) had been displaced forwards, as xrays showed that it had been. Once the tension had been relieved by correcting the deformity the knee swelled rapidly, as is often the case.

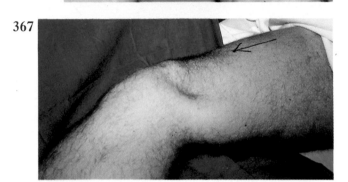

368 Testing anteroposterior glide showed excessive forward movement of the tibia but not obviously more than normal movement backwards, showing that the posterior cruciate ligament was intact.

Comment Testing the anteroposterior movement of the tibia on the femur is a well-known guide to the state of the cruciate ligaments. However, having found the range of movement to be greater than normal, one must ascertain whether the tibia is being pulled forwards out of position, as in this case, or into position because the posterior cruciate ligament has been torn and allows the head of the tibia to be pulled backwards by the hamstrings.

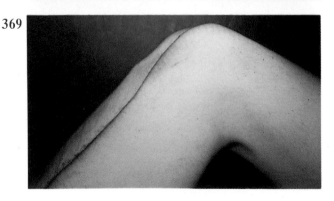

369 The unforced backward sagging of the head of the tibia caused by rupture of the posterior cruciate ligament. Note the mark of impact on the front of the head of the tibia.

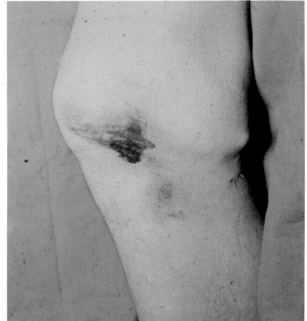

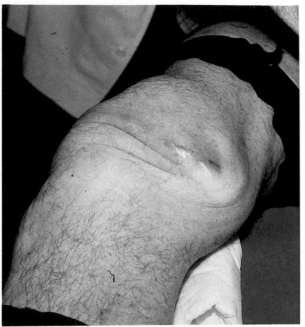

370 An anteromedial view of the right knee. Supracondylar fracture or displacement of the lower epiphysis of the femur can cause striking deformity. When the skin is stretched like this over a bony prominence, manipulation should be carried out as soon as possible.

371 Although subluxation of the knee is rare, it can cause an appearance similar to the foregoing.

The tendo Achillis

372 Rupture of the tendo Achillis can cause a visible dent and a more obvious palpable gap.

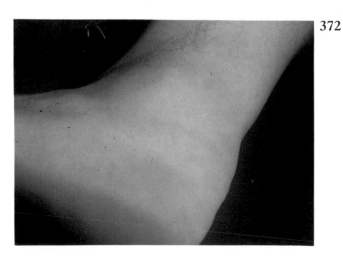

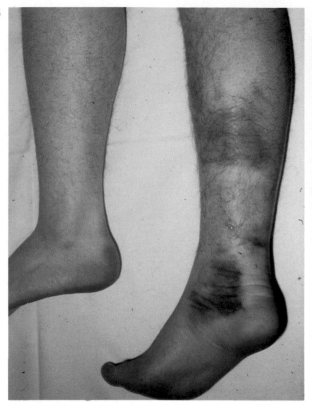

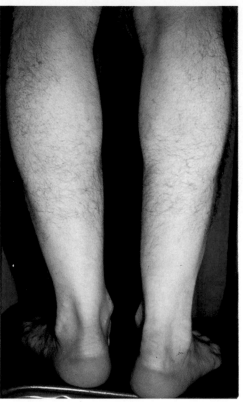

373 Torn muscle. This amount of bruising and swelling after a violent effort to leap or run is much more likely to result from a torn muscle than from a ruptured tendon.

Partial rupture of the tendo Achillis is not a rare diagnosis but the condition may not occur. The diagnosis is tempting when there is no gap and the victim retains quite strong plantar flexion at the ankle. The explanation is that the frayed ends of the ruptured tendon have not been pulled clear of each other and any muscle of which the tendon passes behind one or other of the malleoli can plantar flex the ankle.

374 The different shapes of the two calves are characteristic of previous rupture (on the right side) and persist even after repair has allowed a return to vigorous activities. The most sensitive test of the state of the tendo Achillis is Thompson's. The patient lies prone and the muscles of the affected calf are squeezed firmly from side to side. If slight plantar flexion occurs, the tendon is intact.

Comment The possibility that the tendo Achillis has been ruptured is not always considered. The characteristic event is a violent leap or lunge by either an athletic person or someone past middle-age undertaking unfamiliar exercise; this had been referred to as the 'overeager uncle' syndrome. Following the effort the leg is painful and weak. At the moment of rupture the victim may feel as though something snapped but it is worth asking if he or she thought that the calf had been struck a heavy blow. It is not unusual for a squash player who ruptures the tendon to turn round angrily on his opponent and ask why he did that, to the other player's complete mystification.

7 Ankle and foot

Bruises and grazes

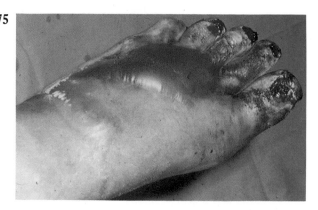

375 Severe and extensive crushing with multiple fractures of the toes, some of which had to be amputated. The severity of the injury was not evident initially. Sometimes the skin under a blood blister or a crust is found to be healthy.

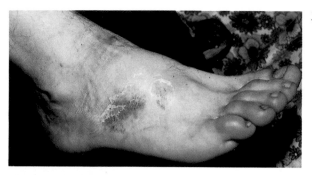

376 This foot was run over by a wheel with a solid rubber tyre. The damage was confined almost entirely to the soft tissues, which healed without grafting.

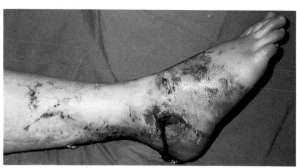

377 This foot was injured in a road accident. Apart from the wound, the appearance was similar to that of the previous case, but there was extensive undermining and an open fracture-dislocation of the talocalcanean and ankle joints. The injuries healed well after exploration, toilet and internal fixation. Good function was regained.

Wounds

Pricks and punctures

When somebody treads on a nail it may pass between the heads of the metatarsals and reach nearly as far as the skin on the dorsum. Fragments of footwear may be carried in; it is best to assume that they have been, regard the wound as infected and treat it accordingly.

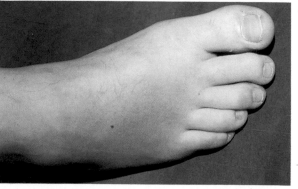

378 If an abscess forms, it may be on the dorsum of the foot and contain the foreign matter, as in this case.

Comment (i) When there is no certainty that foreign matter is present in such a case, immediate exploration is likely to do much more harm than good. (ii) Accidental puncture of the dorsum of the foot with a garden fork is not all that unusual. If the tine of the fork has pierced footwear, the possibility that foreign matter is present should be dealt with in this way.

379

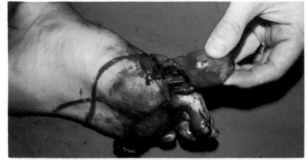

379 A crush injury such as this is tantamount to an amputation, which should be completed surgically. Little more than the tendons needed to be cut.

Comment It is far more useful to the patient if the surgeon ensures prompt healing by removing all tissue of doubtful viability, than to try to preserve all possibly viable tissue. Even in the young and active there are few purposes for which any of the toes are necessary.

380

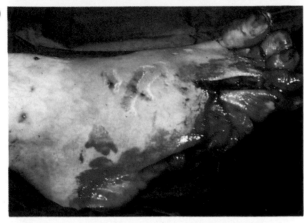

380 A foot that was run over by the wheel of a railway coach. After several attempts to save most of what remained, the youth concerned disappeared with a well-healed Chopart's amputation.

381

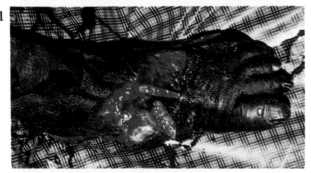

381 The result of a severe crush injury that spared the skin of the heel. In spite of being 65 years of age, the man made a good recovery after an immediate Syme's amputation. The state of the other foot and the accessible arteries suggested that his peripheral circulation was good.

382

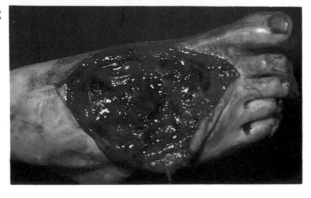

382 A large dorsal wound with multiple fractures of the metatarsals resulted from a road accident. Six weeks later, the foot had nearly healed following immediate internal fixation of the fractures. Skin grafting was carried out when dead dorsal skin was removed after 2 weeks.

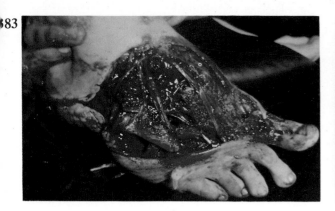

383 This very severe injury was caused when the foot was smashed over the footrest of a motor cycle. The tarsus escaped serious injury but only the medial two metatarsals and toes were worth saving. The man returned to work as a barber.

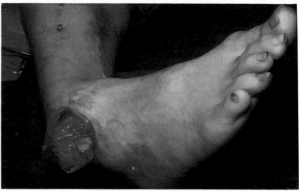

384 The shin bears the marks of a heavy blow that forced the ankle into adduction, tore open the ankle joint and forced the fibula out through the skin. The articular cartilage of the tibia was also exposed. A similar injury can occur at the talocalcanean joint and leave the talus sticking out.

385 A passing vehicle ran over this man's right ankle while he was painting a line on the road with the foot stretched out behind him. The wound went more than half way round the limb. The foot retained a good blood and nerve supply. The lower end of the fibula was comminuted. In such a case, the best prospect for healing of the wound(s) is provided by retaining the foot accurately in position and so keeping tension off the suture line. This required internal fixation. The small fragments of the fibula were held precariously in position with Kirschner's wire but the main protection was provided by driving a Steinmann's pin through the heel and into the tibia until the wound had healed soundly. The main wound looked encouraging a week later and the small incision through intact skin on the outer side healed uneventfully.

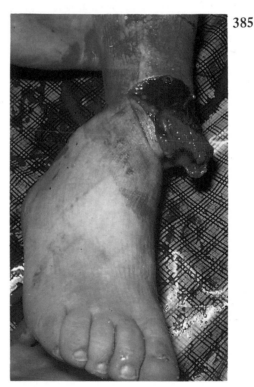

385

Comment The damage done by transfixing joints in this way is negligible compared with that resulting from the injury; once the transfixing device has been removed, useful movement can return. Five years later this man's ankle was stiff and uncomfortable but he was working; 16 years after that he had not returned for further treatment.

Flaying

386

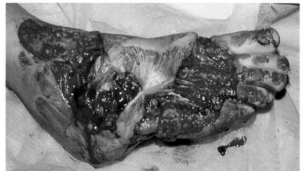

386 A foot that was smashed when the pedal of a girl's bicycle was broken off by a car. The injured limb made a good functional recovery after toilet, internal fixation and delayed primary Thiersch grafting.

Comment The stiffness that is certain to follow serious injuries of the foot is compatible with good function, if the foot is of normal shape. This is best ensured by fixation, usually with Kirschner's wires.

387

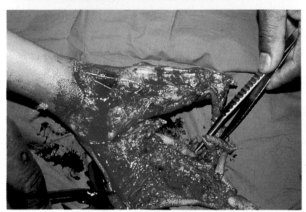

387 Both this girl's feet lost nearly all their skin and some toes when they were run over in the road. The left foot is shown here.

388

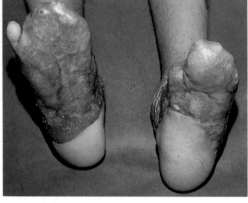

388 Split skin grafts applied after a few days were intact some years later. The child wore soft shoes such as 'trainers' and led an active life at school. This result owed much to the fact that there was normal skin under the heels. Split skin serves well on the soles, if it is not required to take all the weight.

389

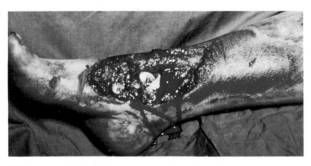

389 A road accident ground away skin, the tendon of tibialis anterior and part of the lower end of the tibia of a 4-year-old girl. The ankle joint was open and the navicular bone was exposed. The wound healed after toilet and split skin grafting. After this she used the extensor muscles of the toes to extend the ankle and because they were no longer balanced by the action of tibialis anterior, they pulled the foot into eversion.

Comment Destruction of the tendons at a child's ankle can have serious and lasting effects upon growth as well as function, unless balanced action of muscles is restored. In this girl's case, until she stopped growing, numerous operations were performed to counteract the deforming effect of damage to the lower epiphysis of the tibia, as well as to restore muscular balance. Twenty-two years later she was leading an active life, in spite of a very stiff and ugly ankle.

Swelling and deformity

The ankle

390 This appearance of an ankle is very frequently seen in any emergency room. It is typical of an injury that occurred a few hours previously. The swelling represents an increase in volume by about half a litre of blood.

Comment If an ankle is seen within an hour or so of being injured the position of the swelling marks the site of injury and the tenderness is also localised accurately. As time passes, the swelling and the tenderness both become more diffuse and clinical diagnosis is less likely to be accurate. It may be argued that if there is a history of injury and the ankle is swollen and painful, it has to be xrayed and that this makes careful clinical examination unnecessary. Some of the following illustrations show that this reasoning is not without dangers.

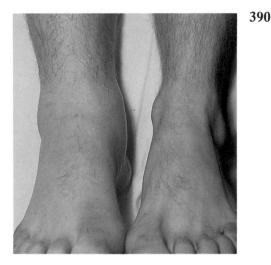

390

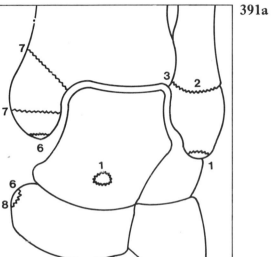

391a

391 a and b These diagrams show the tender places that occur with the more frequent injuries:
1. Sprains, with or without fracture, of the lateral ligament.
2. Spiral fractures of the fibula. Tenderness at the back is of particular significance.
3. Sprains of the anterior inferior tibiofibular ligament and Tillaux's fracture. The tenderness and swelling may extend some way up from here because of associated tearing of the deep fascia.
4. Fracture of the base of the 5th metatarsal bone.
5. Fractures of the lateral wall of the calcaneus.
6. Sprains and sprain-fractures of the medial ligament.
7. Fractures of the medial malleolus.
8. Sprains at the tuberosity of the navicular bone.

It takes only a few seconds to examine these sites and there is no excuse for failing to do so.

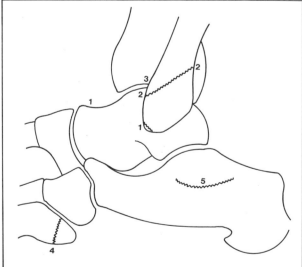

391b

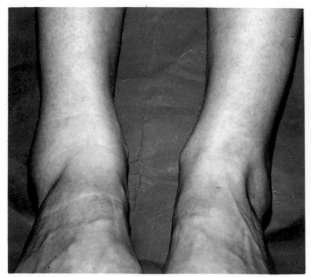

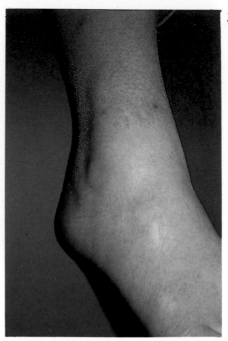

392 The hollows in front of the malleoli had been lost and there was no swelling elsewhere. This suggested an effusion into the ankle and a mild fracture as its cause. With this possibility in mind xray films should therefore be examined with great care. The mild fracture that was present in this case might have been missed but for the warning provided by the clinical evidence of an effusion.

393 There was tenderness over the front of the lateral malleolus with swelling there and a little higher up; the cause was a sprain-fracture of the fibula.

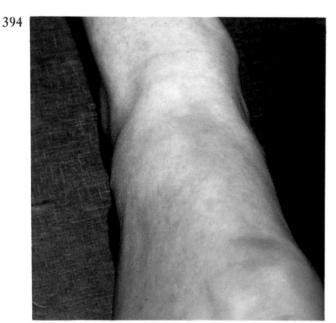

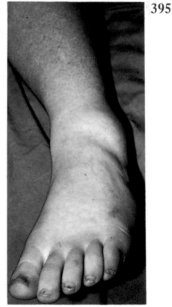

394 The swelling was in the region of the belly of extensor digitorum brevis and appeared to be bounded proximally by the lateral part of the inferior extensor retinaculum; it had tracked up from a sprain-fracture of the front of the calcaneus, near where the retinaculum is attached to it.

395 The patient was a 14-year-old girl who had twisted her ankle. The site of swelling and tenderness was best shown by this view and was over the attachment of the anterior interior tibiofibular ligament to the tibia.

396 A fragment with the amount of displacement shown is worth replacing and, if necessary, fixing surgically.

Comment Tillaux's fracture is rare but usually occurs in girls in their early 'teens. Slight displacement is not worth operating on.

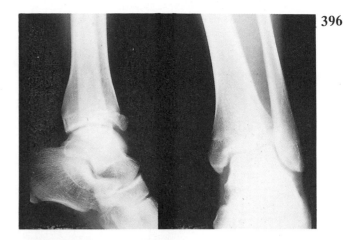

396

397 This patient had twisted his foot. The swelling had spread widely on the lateral side of both the foot and the ankle, but the tender place was at the base of the 5th metatarsal bone, which had been pulled off.

Comment The fact that there is an epiphysis at the base of the 5th metatarsal will not cause confusion if it is remembered that fracture lines are transverse, whereas epiphyseal lines are longitudinal. Rarely, the two conditions occur together.

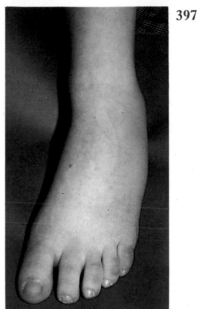

397

398 Such extensive bruising and swelling suggests that there had been a fairly severe injury, but it will be noted that there is no deformity. There was a bad sprain, not a complete rupture of the lateral ligament, and it was a day old.

Comment The patient's account of what happened is not always clear or, though clear, may be misleading. As an example, inversion is an inward twisting of the foot at the talocalcanean or ankle joint, or both, but the patient may describe this movement as the 'ankle going outwards', as in a sense it does.

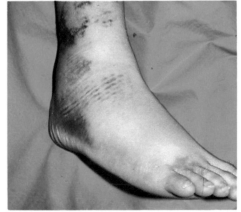

398

Fractures of the calcaneus and some errors and omissions

When a patient says that he has injured his ankle and it is found to be swollen and tender, it is likely that the ankle will be xrayed and the films may be passed as normal, whereas an alert examiner will see that there is a fracture of the calcaneus. If it were customary for the injured 'ankle' to be examined from behind, it is likely that broadening of the heel with swelling and tenderness on its outer side would more often be recognised, and that radiographic attention would be directed at the calcaneus rather than the ankle joint.

399

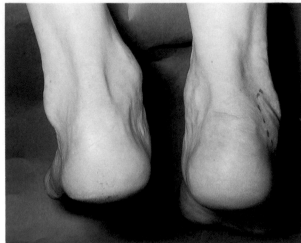

399 In this very mild fracture of the lateral wall of the calcaneus the swelling was at first localised and was most obvious from behind.

400

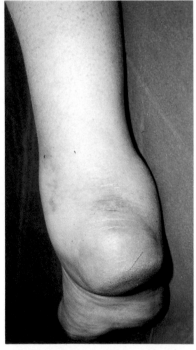

401

400 With more severe fractures of the heel there is obvious swelling on both sides of what could well be called the ankle. In this case there was also the bruising in the sole that often follows this fracture.

401 A severe crush fracture causes obvious displacement as well as swelling and the foot looks flat. Marked swelling is sometimes accompanied by blistering, which may be the result of delay in seeking advice.

Deformity of the ankle

Backward displacement of the foot is a familiar feature of the more severe fracture-dislocations.

402
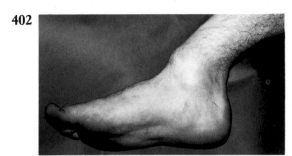

403
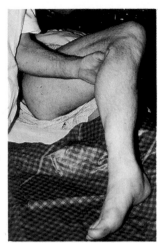

402 This degree of deformity is exceptional and was accompanied by striking lateral rotation of the foot.

403 The deformity was even more obvious when the knee was bent and showed that there was 90 degrees of lateral rotation at the fracture. This appearance is characteristic of the rare condition in which the fibula is displaced so far backwards that it becomes locked behind the tibia. This is not recognised easily from the xray appearance but the following points should be noted.

404
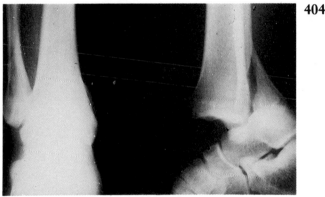

404 (i) The body of the talus appears to be caught on the back edge of the tibia.
(ii) The medial malleolus appears to be level with the back of the tibia, whereas its natural position is near the middle of the shadow of the tibia. Because the film is placed beside the foot for a lateral view of the ankle, when this deformity is present the tibia will be rotated medially in relation to the film but the fibula is not carried forwards with it.

405 B represents a lateral view of the ankle, with the medial malleolus in its natural position and the fibula behind the tibia. **A represents an oblique view of the ankle** that results from placing the film parallel with the foot. The shadows of the tibia and fibula are partly superimposed and the medial malleolus is far back, as in **404**.

405
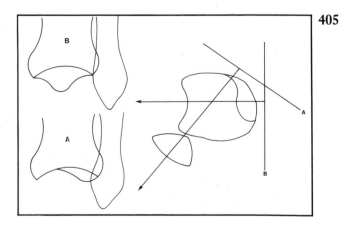

Comment Because the skin is stretched pale on the inner side of the ankle, it may be tempting to try to correct the deformity by what is sometimes optimistically referred to as 'a quick tweak'. In fact, this cannot be done; even when the fibula has been exposed, it requires fairly strong leverage to return it to its rightful place.

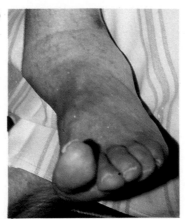

406 In this case the foot had been shifted sideways with little or no twisting. Xrays showed separation of the fibula, which had been broken, from the tibia.

Deformity of the foot

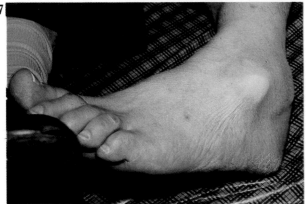

407 A striking example of subtalar dislocation, with the head of the talus stretching the skin, which requires prompt relief. 'A quick tweak' corrected the deformity; after momentary discomfort the patient was much more comfortable. The 'tweak' requires a firm grip on the heel, which is held in the hollow of one hand, and a firm grip with the other hand on the dorsum of the metatarsus. For the left foot, the right hand should hold the heel and vice versa. The foot is pulled downwards in the line of the leg and is twisted outwards (eversion), but without altering the position of the ankle joint. Replacement is not usually difficult but repeated manipulation should not be attempted without general anaesthesia because sometimes tendons slip between the bones and an operation is necessary to extract them.

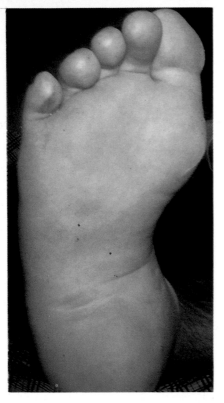

408 and **409** The inward hooking of this man's foot was particularly well seen from below and the accentuation of the plantar arch, with the prominent creasing, from the side. The victim was the driver of a sports car that crashed head-on with another vehicle at an estimated closing speed of about 100 mph. The driver was wearing a seat-belt and only his right foot was injured. This happened because the floor by the pedals was so deeply indented that the foot was trapped between it and a support of the seat, which made an obvious mark on his heel. The resulting longitudinal loading forcibly accentuated the natural arches of the foot and caused a radiologically very complicated combination of fractures of the metatarsals, navicular and talus, with dislocation of the ankle and talocalcaneonavicular joints. In spite of the radiologically complex appearance, the injury was comparable with the previous one and the deformity was quite easily corrected, after which three Kirschner's wires maintained correction. Three years later he sustained a mild fracture of the tibia while skiing; nearly 20 years after the injury the aches and pains in the foot were still not severe enough to prevent him from skiing.

Comment This case, perhaps more than any other, emphasises the fact that stiffness, even of both the foot and the ankle, is compatible with good function if there is no deformity. Recurrence of deformity is best prevented by internal fixation, which allows early movement of the uninjured joints.

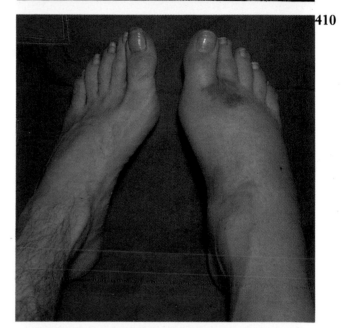

410 The right foot was extensively swollen, including the sole, but it was not obviously deformed. Xrays showed a pattern of tarsometatarsal fractures consistent with less forcible longitudinal loading than in the last case; the arches of the foot had been accentuated, but not so much.

Comment (i) The badly swollen foot has probably been badly injured, but to the inexperienced eye the xray appearances can be reassuringly mild. It is prudent to compare the injured foot with the uninjured foot. It is always wise to seek expert advice within a few hours.
(ii) Although the general patterns of compression-inversion injuries are much the same, the details vary a good deal. They include crushing of the navicular bone against the head of the talus, tarsometatarsal fracture-subluxations and talocalcaneonavicular dislocations.

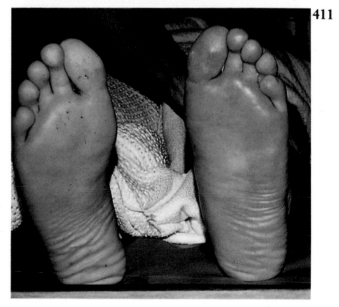

411 In this case the general swelling of the left foot, which was very much like that in 410, was accompanied by loss of the medial concavity. The injury was caused by an abducting force at the tarsometatarsal joints.

Comment (i) This type of injury can be caused by a fall in which the foot as a whole, and not just a toe, has been stubbed.
(ii) In such a case the inexperienced eye may not recognise a gap or a fracture between the bases of the 1st and 2nd metatarsals, the loss of the spaces that are usually shown at some of the joints between tarsal and metatarsal bones, and the fact that the base of the 5th metatarsal bone can be almost level with the front edge of the calcaneus.

Classification

To classify the major injuries of the foot on anatomical grounds is less informative, and less practically useful, than relating the general patterns of the injuries to the forces that have caused them. Inversion or adduction with compression acts at the talocalcaneonavicular joint and neighbouring structures; abduction, usually with compression, acts at the tarsometatarsal joints and eversion can dislocate the talonavicular joint. An injury that is homologous with Bennett's fracture-subluxation also occurs. There is also a rare pattern in which the foot has been forced into flexion near its middle.

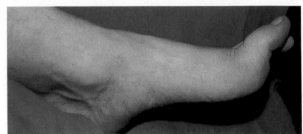

412 This big toe was cocked up because of dislocation of the metatarsophalangeal joint; note the accompanying interphalangeal flexion. This would not occur if there was a fracture of the proximal phalanx.

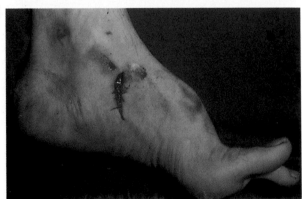

413 Here the big toe was cocked up by the effect of the dorsal hump on the tendon of extensor hallucis longus. Note that the interphalangeal joint was straight. The injury was a fracture-subluxation of the 1st cuneometatarsal joint, which is the homologue of Bennett's injury. The appearance of the foot is characteristic of such an injury.

Infection

Acute haematogenous osteomyelitis in the foot is rare and it may escape diagnosis when it is first seen in its early stages.

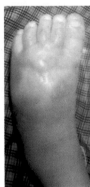 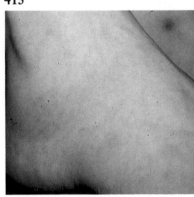

414 Metatarsal osteomyelitis. In this case there had been several days' delay in seeking treatment for osteomyelitis of the 1st metatarsal bone.

415 Early osteomyelitis of the calcaneus.

Comment Osteomyelitis should be thought of when, usually, a child complains of pain coming on only several hours after a blow or wrench. Apart from local tenderness, initially there is little to find that is abnormal and a bruise or sprain may be diagnosed, but with these the symptoms and signs are present within the first few hours. If early osteomyelitis is suspected, the child should be rested and observed closely. An antibiotic should be given if there has been no improvement after 6-12 hours.

8 Multiple injuries

Many of the injuries that have already been shown have not occurred in isolation and some of their contributions to diagnosis in the case of multiple injuries have been indicated. Their appearances are often at least as informative in the severely injured and uncommunicative as when a detailed history is available. An experienced eye cast over a severely injured person recently arrived in hospital will often identify much useful information. There are patterns of injury that are characteristic of particular sorts of accident and when one or more components of a pattern are observed, others should be sought.

Experience has taught that examination of the seriously injured should be carried out systematically from head to foot, back and front and not system by system; that the injuries that are likely to be present as a result of the accident should be deliberately looked for and that the injuries that are liable to be overlooked should also be looked for in the same way. Remember that stab wounds and bullet wounds are sometimes both multiple and widespread.

This chapter deals mostly with patterns of injury and their interpretation; most are the results of road accidents and other causes of great violence.

Road accidents

Pedestrians

Most pedestrians are struck from the side. Children are usually struck on the right side, because they have run out in front of a vehicle, whereas old persons are often hit from the left as they approach the far side of the road. The pattern of injuries inflicted is also influenced by the height of the impact. A pedestrian who is struck below the centre of gravity is thrown into the air and may land on the bonnet or even penetrate the windscreen. This can result in other injuries and these tend also to be on the side of the original impact. If the impact is above the centre of gravity, the victim is thrown away from the vehicle and the injuries caused by that impact are often accompanied by injuries on the other side as a result of impact with the road.

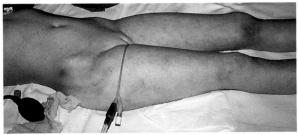

416 Primary impact was on the right side of the pelvis and this little girl's legs. There was a mild fracture of the pelvis and a rupture of the kidney.

417 and **418 In the same patient secondary impact with the road caused these injuries of the loin and face and also fatal damage to the brain.**

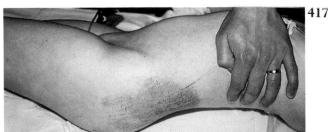

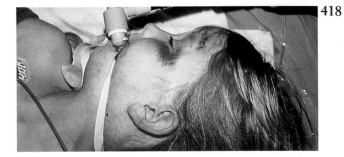

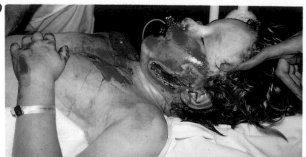

419 The wounds over the jaw, chest and hand were friction burns that occurred when the child was trapped under a bus. There were also a fracture of the pelvis and mild injuries of the abdominal organs.

Motor-cyclists

Many riders sustain the primary injury when the right side is struck by an on-coming vehicle. Secondary injuries can result from being thrown from the motor-cycle, and perhaps into the path of a third vehicle, or because the machine falls on to the rider's left leg.

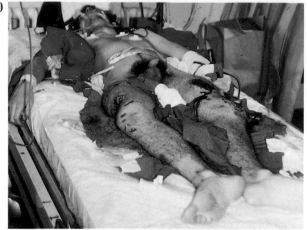

420 An all-too-familiar sight late at night at a weekend. There were severe open fractures of the femora. The pupils were already dilating and reacting sluggishly; the veins were empty and the belly was distended. Marks of impact on the chest suggested rupture of the aorta and damage to the heart, which were not confirmed. Attempts at resuscitation were abandoned after the patient had received blood equivalent in quantity to his own blood volume. Necropsy revealed severe ruptures of the liver and spleen.

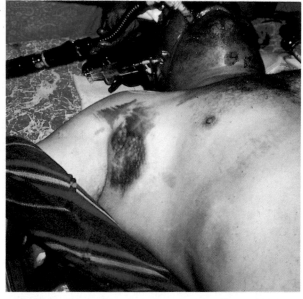

421 Swelling of this size shortly after the accident suggested that a large artery had been torn. The patient died and there was no necropsy.

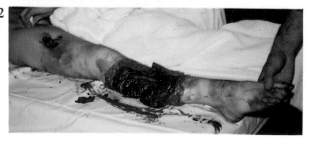

422 The marks of primary impact on the right lower limb. There were also signs of secondary impact on the left leg.

423 An open fracture of the femur in which the bone had pierced the trousers and had been stripped of all soft tissue for about 6 inches. In such a case, road dirt may have been driven into the marrow cavity.

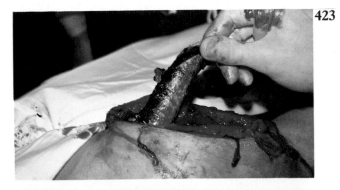

424 There was also a severe open and comminuted fracture of the tibia and fibula, with a wide gap between the two bones. The foot was bloodless as well as having the skin torn from the heel. The leg was amputated below the knee and the stump, as well as the wound in the thigh, was sewn up 3 days later, when the femur was fixed with a Küntscher's nail. In the absence of other injuries, the youth went home 6 days after his accident and made an uninterrupted recovery. His pillion passenger sustained similar injuries but did not have to lose his leg; he was treated in much the same way as the driver but developed infection around the nail in his thigh.

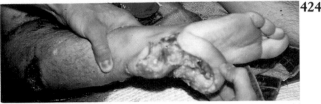

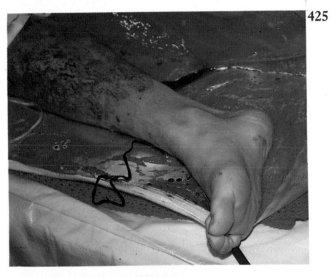

425 When the pillion passenger reached hospital he was pale and cold all over and there were no pulses to be felt at either ankle. It is fitting that the serious injuries of the right lower limb should be dressed and splinted without delay but the limb was not forgotten. As the rest of the patient regained warmth and colour in his skin, it was noted that the right foot also recovered. Unless the possibility of damage to an artery is kept in mind in such circumstances, it could easily go unrecognised in the process of dealing with the rest of the patient and with the limb temporarily out of the limelight.

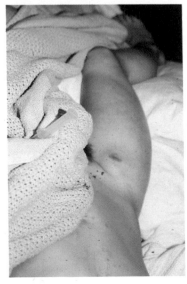

426 There were closed fractures just below the right hip and the right knee. A graze on the chest might have resulted from the primary impact or from the rider's subsequent passage through a hedge, some of which accompanied him to hospital.

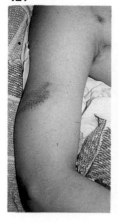 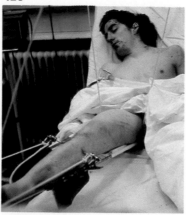

427 A blow on the right arm damaged the radial nerve; there was also a traction lesion of the brachial plexus on the same side.

428 Injuries of the left thigh and brachial plexus were accompanied by unconsciousness for some days. The bruising at the root of the neck will be noted (*see* also **12**).

Paralysis in the uncommunicative patient

The possibility that paralysis of spinal or other origin is present in a casualty that is unconscious or otherwise uncommunicative has been referred to; it deserves further consideration.

The most important aid to diagnosis is to recognise the possibility. The evidence to support the possibility should then be sought. It includes the following:

Warning signs 1 Wounds, bruises and other evidence of injury in the course of a nerve (*see* **12, 148, 331, 427, 428**).
2 Fractures and dislocations near nerves, for example, of the zygoma, spine, shoulder, humerus, elbow, hip and knee.

3 Marks of injury of the face and brow in persons past middle-age (*see* **9**).
4 Low blood pressure in a person who is warm, pink, alert and not sweating (*see* **2** below). The output of urine is not reduced.

Supporting evidence 1 Loss of tone, reflexes and spontaneous or reactive movements of one or more limbs.
2 Loss of sweating. Except on the fingers, where the difference between dryness and the natural moisture of the skin is fairly easy to recognise by touch, natural sweating is often imperceptible. When the casualty is sweating, areas where it is absent should be sought.
3 Other evidence of sympathetic paralysis (*see* **27**).

429 In this man it could be seen that the right upper lid was drooping and on close examination the right pupil was smaller and less reactive to light than the left. He had suffered fracture-dislocation of the spine and was tetraplegic; spinal paralysis is not necessarily symmetrical.

4 Posture

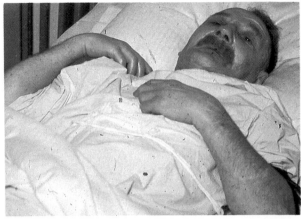

430 This shows the characteristic posture with a lesion of the spine at C6-C7. A lesion at C5-C6 causes the upper limbs to adopt the 'hands up' position.

5 The pattern of breathing that occurs when only the diaphragm is acting (*see* **108**).

6 If a casualty is deeply unconscious, a finger passed down the throat may feel a gap, boggy swelling or abnormal movement of the spine that occurs with hyperextension injuries in young persons. Xray films may be passed as normal because they show no fracture or dislocation; that is because the lesion affects the intervertebral disc. However, there may be thickening of the prevertebral soft tissues; that is not conclusive but it is a useful warning.

7 Priapism.

8 The presence of the anal and bulbocavernosus reflexes.

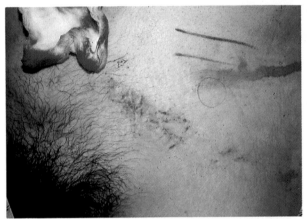

431 The injuries of the head and face suggested head-on impact (*see* **66**) but this mark across the left groin looked as though it had been caused by the passage of a wheel over the limb as a secondary injury.

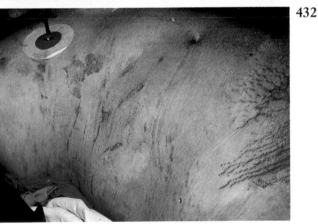

432 It was reported that this young motor-cyclist had been found under the wheel of an articulated lorry. The marks on his trunk were consistent with such a mishap. There were severe injuries of the pelvis and abdominal organs. A wound in the groin extended into the buttock and loin, where there was extensive undermining.

When the victim reached hospital he was restless and confused. However, when he had received 7 bags of blood, his brain was fully oxygenated and his mind was clear. He had not been injured above his costal margin. Hypoxia of the brain is a treatable cause of impaired consciousness (*see* **10** and **11**).

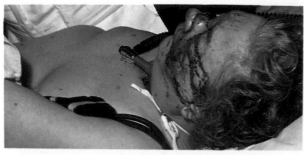

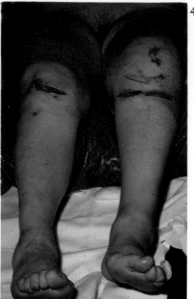

433 and 434 This female driver was not wearing a seat-belt and had a characteristic pattern of injuries comprising a stove-in chest and fractures of the thighs and ankles, as well as these injuries of the knees.

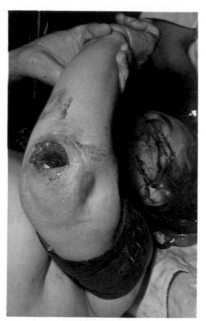

435 There was also a wound of the elbow that entered the joint through a fracture of the olecranon process of the ulna.

Comment The injuries in this case included most of the consequences of forcible impact with the windscreen, steering wheel, dashboard and floor. Given sufficient deformation of the vehicle, such injuries might occur even in a properly restrained person.

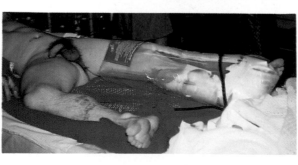

436 The position of the right lower limb may suggest anterior dislocation of the hip but it will be noted that the thigh was swollen; there was a fracture of the femur. The hip was xrayed and was found to be normal. There was also an open fracture of the left leg. This man occupied the front passenger seat in a car and suffered a ruptured spleen and a haematoma of the mesentery (*see* also **80** and **81**).

437 A head-on crash caused coma and multiple fractures of ribs, from which surgical emphysema spread widely in the neck and chest and then into the peritoneal cavity. There was no damage below the diaphragm.

Comment The fact that air can reach the peritoneal cavity in this way has long been known but it is not widely known. In the unconscious victim with severe injuries of the chest it may be impossible to rule out perforation of the gut without resorting to laparotomy.

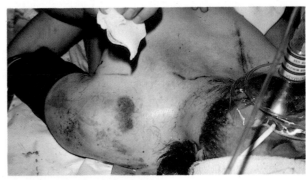

Complicating head injury

Unconsciousness can complicate diagnosis but restless confusion can greatly increase the difficulties of treating fractures; fortunately this is unusual.

438 An elderly man sustained a stove-in forehead and a fracture of the fibula with a large flap over the shin. In spite of what did not seem to be very secure fixation, it withstood his blundering efforts to get up and walk and nearly all the overlying flap survived.

Restless hands can be as detrimental to splints and dressings as can be general restlessness. Physical restraint should, if possible, be avoided because it can aggravate restlessness.

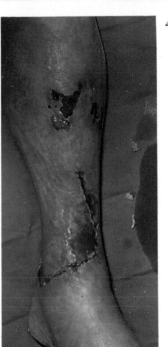

Industrial accidents

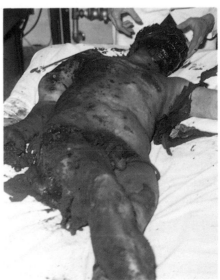

439 The result of an explosion that had the effect of blackening the victim. The right hand had been shattered and the right thigh had been flayed extensively and also pulped. The man died during attempts at resuscitation.

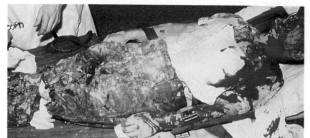

440

440 In spite of the comparably alarming appearance when this man reached hospital after a furnace that he had been repairing collapsed on him, he had suffered little physical injury (*see* **167**).

Wilful injury

Children

Characteristically, wilful injuries in children are multiple. There may be plausible explanations for some of the injuries, but the mien and behaviour of the victim may arouse suspicion even when the parents' account invites acceptance.

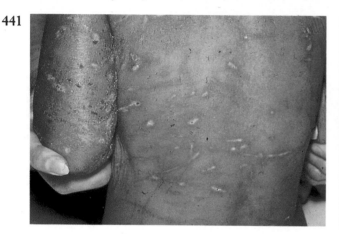

441

441 There is no blameless explanation for such scars, some of which result from cigarette burns.

442

442 Whatever reasons may be given for the numerous scars on this boy, there is only one explanation for the imprint of a rubber heel on the abdominal wall.

Alleged assault

One of the emergency room officer's most difficult tasks can be to decide whether injuries took place before or after a plaintiff was taken into police custody, and to establish how the injuries were caused. Whenever possible, the responsibility should be accepted by an experienced doctor but if this is not possible—and it should be remembered that the sooner the findings are recorded the better—a junior doctor must carry out this important task.

Useful rules are:

1 Get as much detail as possible about how the injuries are alleged to have occurred and record it carefully.

2 Carry out a very thorough physical examination of the patient, not just the injuries, and record the findings in full. It is also wise to record ones opinion whether or not injuries are consistent with the allegations. In some cases it may be possible to state that the injury was certainly caused as alleged, but junior hospital staff will be wise to err on the side of caution in this respect. An opinion about consistency is easier to defend than a confident statement of cause.

3 Photograph all marks of injury.

4 Xray any areas in which there is evidence of injury, because a normal looking bone may later show changes such as subperiosteal calcification of local rarefaction that support a history of injury.

443 This mark over the sacroiliac joint is consistent with a blow by a fist, boot, stick or in the course of a fall or legitimate struggle. What did cause it cannot be stated with any assurance of being right.

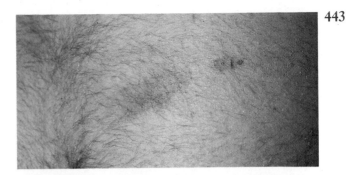

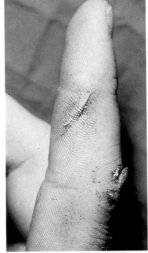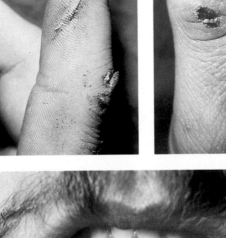

444 and 445 The marks on these fingers are more consistent with a punch having been thrown or their being barked in a struggle than with an alleged bite.

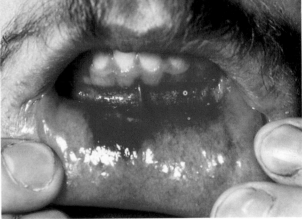

446 Bruising on the inner surface of the lip is consistent with a blow that was more likely to be deliberate than accidental.

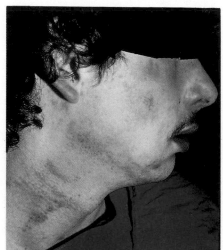

447 The marks on the face are consistent with having been made by blows and those on the neck by a blow or a firm grip.

448

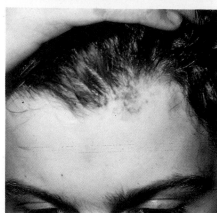

448 There is nothing about this mark to indicate what made it.

449

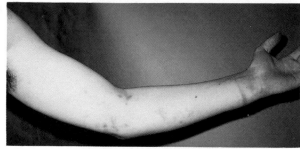

449 The marks on this limb could have been caused during a struggle.

450

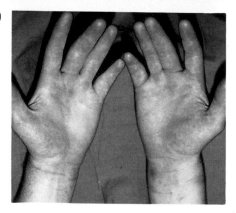

450 The marks of handcuffs on the radial rather than the ulnar sides of the wrists are consistent with efforts to ward off blows, but could have been caused in other ways.

During examination-in-chief and cross-examination the medical witness should pay very careful attention to the wording of both the questions asked and the answers given. The witness should remember that his/her task is usually to assist the Court in coming to a decision and not try to make the decision for the Court.

Index